Welcome...

Kundalini

Yoga

The Shakti Path to Soul Awakening

Original title "Kundalini Yoga"
by Sri Swami Sivananda Saraswati

Translated by

Lateef Terrell Warnick

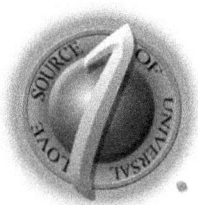

Hardback: 978-1-939199-12-6
Paperback: 978-1-939199-13-3
ebook: 978-1-939199-14-0
Library of Congress Control Number: 2012918912

Kundalini Yoga: The Shakti Path to Soul Awakening

1. Religion/ Spirituality 2. Mind, Body & Spirit 3. Mysticism 4. Metaphysics 5. New Age 6. Self-Help 7. Warnick, Lateef Terrell I. Title

Printed in the United States of America

Dedicated to man's eternal quest to reunite with the Source of all Light and the gurus who help to dispel the darkness along the way!

*"When the soul sees itself as a Center
surrounded by its circumference, when the
Sun knows that it is a Sun, surrounded by its
whirling planets - then is it ready for the
Wisdom and Power of the Masters"*

1 S.O.U.L. | Self-Awakened
Spiritual Network, Life Coaching & Non Profit Org

Be sure to share your thoughts, feedback and reviews with us
online and on social media. Also meet like-minds and find more
on spiritual books, yoga, ayurveda, reiki, metaphysics, mysticism,
enlightenment, meditation, holistic living, universal love,
esotericism and self-realization at www.selfawakened.com

Table of Contents

Kundalini Yoga: The Shakti Path to Soul Awakening

FOREWORD

"The only thing that doesn't change is change itself." At least, in this world of duality that we live in that may be true. However, there are those that have proclaimed that there is a Source to all of life that is eternal and changeless! As long as we are identified with all the transient things of creation, we tend to simply float along as well in this never-ending process of change. Yet if we are able to access the true nature of our souls, we will find that we can transcend this continuously evolving and changing manifestation.

The yogis of ancient times have proclaimed the path to transcending this plane of relativity to access the realm of the Absolute is through yoga. Yoga means the union of soul and Spirit. Yoga is the means, process and techniques for union and also the state of union. Yet, the Truth Seeker starting out on his spiritual quest may be overwhelmed with the seemingly various types of yoga. Hence, as founder of 1 S.O.U.L. Publishing, I have made the efforts to disseminate greater awareness of written works expounding on the essence of yoga. Part of 1 S.O.U.L.'s mantra is "Many rivers... One Ocean; many branches... One Tree; many paths... One Destination; many stories... One Truth!"

This means that, ultimately, all religions and even the atheistic path of the skeptic will lead the sincere seeker to the same Self-Realization. And among those who may practice the various paths of yoga, they are merely different petals of the same flower. There are numerous types of yoga. Throughout this series we will focus on the more popular ones being Raja, Jnani, Karma, Bhakti, Hatha and Kundalini. Again, it is not important to try to "rank" the various types because no one path is better than another rather each path may be more suitable for the individual. If a particular path of yoga resonates with you then you should "adopt" it and make sincere efforts to put the techniques into practice.

What you will find in time is that various aspects of all the paths are similar and the closer you get to realizing your Truth, the clearer you will see from your elevated position that you are climbing One Mountain. At the "peak" of Samadhi, the meditator, the meditation and the Source meditated upon become One! Many adepts throughout the ages have defined different aspects of this union from different perspectives. Some define this state of one that has overcome the sense of limitation, separation, avidya or ignorance as samadhi, moksha, kaivalya, soul awakening, self-realization, soul liberation, spiritual enlightenment and so forth. In this series, we creatively describe in flowery terms the various paths with different names but have no confusion – the ultimate goal is the same for all. Raja is considered the "royal" path. Bhakti is the devotional path; Jnani is the path of wisdom, Karma the path of service, Hatha the path of purification and Kundalini the path of shakti. There are other popular types such as Kriya and Laya, which are equally as suitable and can be researched for yourself.

We hope you enjoy this series and, most importantly, practice some of the techniques for merely studying and knowing the paths are not important if you don't make the effort to travel the path! "Namaste" means the Spirit in me salutes the Spirit in you! We wish you many blessings along your journey to your personal attainment to "know thyself" while simultaneously understanding that

"The greatest service you can render unto the world is your own Self-Realization!" Ramana Maharishi

Lateef Terrell Warnick
Author and Founder of 1 S.O.U.L.

PRAYER TO MOTHER KUNDALINI

Wake up Mother Kundalini. Thou whose nature is Bliss Eternal — The Bliss of Brahman. Thou dwelling like a serpent asleep at the lotus of Muladhara, Sore, affected and distressed am I in body and mind, Do thou bless me and leave thy place at the basic lotus. Consort of Siva the Self-caused Lord of Universe, Do thou take thy upward course through the central canal. Leaving behind Svadhishthana, Manipuraka, Anahata, Vishuddha, and Ajna. Be thou united with Siva, thy Lord the God. At Sahasrara— the thousand-petaled-lotus in the brain. Sport there freely, O Mother, Giver of Bliss Supreme. Mother, who is Existence, Knowledge, Bliss Absolute.

Wake up, Mother Kundalini! Wake up.

Chapter One

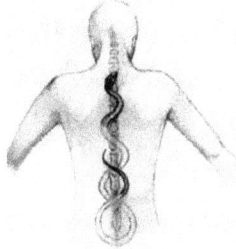

Essence Of Kundalini Yoga

The word YOGA comes from the root Yuj which means to join, and in its spiritual sense, it is that process by which the human spirit is brought into near and conscious communion with, or is merged in, the Divine Spirit, according as the nature of the human spirit is held to be separate from (Dvaita, Visishtadvaita) or one with (Advaita) the Divine Spirit. As, according to Vedanta, the latter proposition is affirmed; Yoga is that process by which the identity of the two (Jivatman and Paramatman)—which identity ever exists, in fact—is realized by the Yogin or practitioner of Yoga. It is so realized because the Spirit has then pierced through the veil of Maya, which as mind and matter obscures this knowledge from itself.

The means by which this is achieved is the Yoga process, which liberates the Jiva from Maya. So the Gheranda-Samhita says: "There is no bond equal in strength to Maya, and no power greater to destroy that bond than Yoga." From an Advaitic or Monistic standpoint, Yoga in the sense of a final union is inapplicable, for union implies a dualism of the Divine and human spirit. In such case, it denotes the *process* rather than the result. When the two are regarded as distinct, Yoga may apply to both. A person who practices Yoga is called a Yogin. All are not competent to attempt Yoga; only a very few are. One must, in this or in other lives, have gone through Karma or selfless service and ritualistic observances, without attachment to the actions or their fruits, and Upasana or devotional worship, and obtained the fruit thereof, viz., a pure mind (Chittasuddhi).

This does not mean merely a mind free from sexual impurity. The attainment of this and other qualities is the A B C of Sadhana. A person may have a pure mind in this sense, and yet be wholly incapable of Yoga. Chittasuddhi consists not merely in moral purity of every kind, but in knowledge, detachment, and capacity for pure intellectual functioning, attention, meditation and so forth. When by Karma Yoga and Upasana, the mind is brought to this point and when, in the case of Jnana Yoga, there is dispassion and detachment from the world and its desires, then the Yoga path is open for the realization of the ultimate Truth. Very few persons indeed are competent for Yoga in its higher form. The majority should seek their advancement along the path of Karma Yoga and devotion.

There are four main forms of Yoga, according to one school of thought, namely Mantra Yoga, Hatha Yoga, Laya Yoga and Raja Yoga; Kundalini Yoga is really Laya Yoga. There is another classification: Jnana Yoga, Raja Yoga, Laya Yoga, Hatha Yoga and Mantra Yoga. This is based on the idea that there are five aspects of spiritual life: - Dharma, Kriya, Bhava, Jnana and Yoga; Mantra Yoga being said to be of two kinds according as it is pursued along the path of Kriya or Bhava. There are seven Sadhanas of Yoga, namely Sat-Karma, Asana, Mudra, Pratyahara, Pranayama, Dhyana and Samadhi, which are cleansing of the body, seat postures for Yoga purposes, the abstraction of the senses from their objects, breath-control, meditation, and ecstasy which is of two kinds—imperfect (Savikalpa) in which dualism is not wholly overcome, and perfect (Nirvikalpa) which is complete Monistic experience–the realization of the Truth of the Mahavakya AHAM BRAHMASMI—a knowledge in the sense of realization which, it is to be observed, does not produce Liberation (Moksha) but is Liberation itself. The Samadhi of Laya Yoga is said to be Savikalpa Samadhi and that of complete Raja Yoga is said to be Nirvikalpa Samadhi. The first four processes are physical, last three mental and supramental. By these seven processes respectively certain qualities are gained, namely, purity (Sodhana), firmness and strength (Dridhata), fortitude (Sthirata), steadiness (Dhairya), lightness (Laghava), realization (Pratyaksha) and detachment leading to Liberation (Nirliptatva).

What is known as the eight-limbed Yoga (Ashtanga Yoga) contains five of the above Sadhanas (Asana, Pranayama, Pratyahara, Dhyana and Samadhi) and three others, namely, Yama or self-control by way of chastity, temperance, avoidance of harm (Ahimsa), and other virtues; Niyama or religious observances, charity and so forth, with devotion to the Lord (Isvara-Pranidhana); and Dharana, the fixing of the internal organ on its object as directed in the Yoga-practice.

Man is a microcosm (Kshudra Brahmanda). Whatever exists in the outer universe exists in him. All the Tattvas and worlds are within him and so is the Supreme Siva-Sakti. The body may be divided into two main parts, namely, the head and trunk on the one hand, and the legs on the other. In man, the center of the body is between these two, at the base of the spine where the legs begin. Supporting the trunk and throughout the whole body there is the spinal cord. This is the axis of the body, just as Mount

Meru is the axis of the earth. Hence, man's spine is called Merudanda, the Meru or axis-staff. The legs and feet are gross which show less signs of consciousness than the trunk with its spinal white and gray matter; which trunk itself is greatly subordinate in this respect to the head containing the organ of mind, or physical brain, with its white and gray matter. The positions of the white and gray matter in the head and spinal column respectively are reversed. The body and legs below the center are the seven lower or nether worlds upheld by the sustaining Sakti or Powers of the universe. From the center upwards, consciousness more freely manifests through the spinal and cerebral centers. Here there are the seven upper regions or Lokas, a term which means "What are seen" (Lokyante), that is, experienced, and are hence the fruits of Karma in the form of particular rebirth. These regions, namely, Bhuh, Bhuvah, Svah, Tapa, Jana, Maha and Satya Lokas correspond with the six centers; five in the trunk, the sixth in the lower cerebral center; and the seventh in the upper brain or Satyaloka, the abode of the Supreme Siva-Sakti.

The six centers are: the Muladhara or root-support situated at the base of the spinal column in a position midway in the perineum between the root of the genitals and the anus; above it, in the region of the genitals, abdomen, heart, chest and throat, and in the forehead between the two eyes, are the Svadhishthana, Manipura, Anahata, Visuddha and Ajna Chakras or lotuses respectively. These are the chief centers, though some texts speak of others such as the Lalana and Manas and Soma Chakras. The seventh region beyond the Chakras is the upper brain, the highest center of manifestation of consciousness in the body and therefore, the abode of the Supreme Siva-Sakti. When it is said to be the "abode", it is not meant that the Supreme is there placed in the sense of our "placing", namely, it is there and not elsewhere! The Supreme is never localized, whilst its manifestations are. It is everywhere both within and without the body, but it is said to be in the Sahasrara, because it is there that the Supreme Siva-Sakti is realized.

And, this must be so, because consciousness is realized by entering in and passing through the higher manifestation of mind, the Sattvamayi Buddhi, above and beyond which is Chit and Chidrupini Saktis themselves. From their Siva-Sakti Tattva aspect are evolved Mind in its form as Buddhi, Ahamkara, Manas and associated senses (Indriyas) the center of which is above the Ajna Chakra and below the Sahasrara. From Ahamkara proceed the Tanmatras, or generals of the sense-particulars, which evolve the five forms of sensible matter (Bhuta), namely, Akasa (ether), Vayu (air), Agni (fire), Apah (water) and Prithvi (earth). The English translation given does not imply that the Bhutas are the same as the English elements of air, fire, water, and earth. The terms indicate varying degrees of matter from the ethereal to the solid. Thus Prithvi or earth is any matter in the Prithvi state; that is, which may be sensed by the Indriya of smell. Mind and matter pervade the whole body. But there are centers therein in which they are predominant. Thus Ajna is the center of mind, and the five lower Chakras are the centers of the five Bhutas; Visuddha of Akasa, Anahata of Vayu, Manipura of Agni, Svadhishthana of Apah, and Muladhara of Prithvi.

In short, man as a microcosm is the all-pervading Spirit (which most purely manifests in the Sahasrara) vehicled by Sakti in the form of mind and matter, the centers of which are the sixth and following five Chakras respectively.

The six Chakras have been identified with the following plexuses commencing from the lowest, the Muladhara; the sacrococcygeal plexus, the sacral plexus, the solar plexus, (which forms the great junction of the right and left sympathetic chains Ida and Pingala with the cerebro-spinal axis). Connected with this is the lumbar plexus. Then follows the cardiac plexus (Anahata), laryngeal plexus, and lastly the Ajna or cerebellum with its two lobes. Above this is the Manas-Chakra or middle cerebrum, and finally, the Sahasrara or upper cerebrum. The six Chakras themselves are vital centers within the spinal column in the white and gray matter there. They may, however, and probably do, influence and govern the gross tract outside the spine in the bodily region lateral to, and co-extensive with, that section of the spinal column in which a particular center is situated. The Chakras are centers of Sakti as vital force. In other words these are centers of Pranasakti manifested by Pranavayu in the living body, the presiding Devatas of which are names for the Universal Consciousness as It manifests in the form of those centers. The Chakras are not perceptible to the gross senses. Even if they were perceptible in the living body, which they help to organize, they disappear with the disintegration of organism at death. Just because post-mortem examination of the body does not reveal these Chakras in the spinal column, some people think that these Chakras do not exist at all, and are merely the fabrication of a fertile brain. This attitude reminds us of a doctor who declared that he had performed many post-mortems and had never yet discovered a soul!

The petals of the lotuses vary, being 4, 6, 10, 12, 16 and 2 respectively, commencing from the Muladhara and ending with Ajna. There are 50 in all, as are the letters of the alphabet, which are in the petals; that is, the Matrikas are associated with the Tattvas; since both are products of the same creative Cosmic process manifesting either as physiological or psychological function. It is noteworthy that the number of the petals is that of the letters leaving out either Ksha or the second La, and that these 50 multiplied by 20 are in the 1000 petals of the Sahasrara, a number which is indicative of infinitude.

But why, it may be asked, do the petals vary in number? Why, for instance, are there 4 in the Muladhara and 6 in the Svadhishthana? The answer given is that the number and position of the Nadis or Yoga-nerves around that Chakra determine the number of petals in any Chakra. Thus, four Nadis surrounding and passing through the vital movements of the Muladhara Chakra, give it the appearance of a lotus of four petals, which are thus configurations made, by the positions of Nadis at any particular center. These Nadis are not those, which are known to the Vaidya. The latter are gross physical nerves. But the former, here spoken of, are called Yoga-Nadis and are subtle channels (Vivaras) along which the Pranic currents flow. The term Nadi comes from the root Nad which means motion. The body is filled with an uncountable number of Nadis. If they were revealed to the eye, the body would present the appearance of a highly complicated chart of ocean currents. Superficially the water seems one and the same. But examination shows that it is moving with varying degrees of force in all directions. All these lotuses exist in the spinal columns.

The Merudanda is the vertebral column. Western anatomy divides it into five regions; and it is to be noted in corroboration of the theory here expounded that these correspond with the regions in which the five Chakras are situated. The central spinal system comprises the brain or encephalon contained within the skull (in which are the

7

Lalana, Ajna, Manas, Soma Chakras and the Sahasrara) as also the spinal cord extending from the upper border of the Atlas below the cerebellum and descending to the second lumbar vertebra where it tapers to a point called the filum terminale. Within the spine is the cord, a compound of gray and white brain matter, in which are the five lower Chakras. It is noteworthy that the filum terminale was formerly thought to be a mere fibrous cord, an unsuitable vehicle, one might think, for the Muladhara Chakra and Kundalini Sakti. More recent microscopic investigations have, however, disclosed the existence of highly sensitive gray matter in the filum terminale, which represents the position of the Muladhara. According to Western science, the spinal cord is not merely a conductor between the periphery and the centers of sensation and volition, but is also an independent center or group of centers. The Sushumna is a Nadi in the center of the spinal column. Its base is called Brahma-Dvara or Gate of Brahman.

As regards the physiological relations of the Chakras all that can be said with any degree of certainty is that the four above Muladhara have relation to the genito-excretory, digestive, cardiac and respiratory functions and that the two upper centers, the Ajna (with associated Chakras) and the Sahasrara denote various forms of its cerebral activity ending in the repose of Pure Consciousness therein gained through Yoga. The Nadis of each side Ida and Pingala are the left and right sympathetic cords crossing the central column from one side to the other, making at the Ajna with the Sushumna a threefold knot called Triveni; which is said to be the spot in the Medulla where the sympathetic cords join together and whence they take their origin—these Nadis together with the two lobed Ajna and the Sushumna forming the figure of the Caduceus of the God Mercury which is said by some to represent them.

How is it that the rousing of Kundalini Sakti and Her union with Siva effect the state of ecstatic union (Samadhi) and spiritual experience which is alleged?

In the first place, there are two main lines of Yoga, namely, Dhyana or Bhavana-Yoga and Kundalini Yoga; and there is a marked difference between the two. The first class of Yoga is that in which ecstasy (Samadhi) is obtained by intellective processes (Kriya-Jnana) of meditation and the like, with the aid, it may be, of auxiliary processes of Mantra or Hatha Yoga (other than the rousing of Kundalini) and by detachment from the world; the second stands apart as that portion of Hatha Yoga in which, though intellective processes are not neglected, the creative and sustaining Sakti of the whole body is actually and truly united with the Lord Consciousness. The Yogin makes Her introduce him to Her Lord, and enjoys the bliss of union through her. Though it is he who arouses Her, it is She who gives knowledge or Jnana, for She is Herself that. The Dhyana Yogin gains what acquaintance with the Supreme state his own meditative powers can give him and knows not the enjoyment of union with Siva in and through the fundamental Body-power.

The two forms of Yoga differ both as to method and result. The Hatha Yogin regards his Yoga and its fruit as the highest; the Jnana Yogin may think similarly of his own. Kundalini is so renowned that many seek to know her. Having studied the theory of this Yoga, one may ask: "Can one get on without it?" The answer is: "It depends upon what you are looking for". If you want to rouse Kundalini Sakti, to enjoy the bliss of union of Siva and Sakti through Her, and to gain the accompanying powers (Siddhis), it is obvious that only the Kundalini Yoga can achieve this end.

In that case, there are some risks incurred. But if Liberation is sought without desire for union through Kundalini, then, such Yoga is not necessary; for, Liberation may be obtained by Pure Jnana Yoga through detachment, the exercise and then the stilling of the mind, without any rousing of the central Bodily-power at all.

Instead of setting out in and from the world to unite with Siva, the Jnana Yogin, to attain this result, detaches himself from the world. The one is the path of enjoyment and the other of asceticism. Samadhi may also be obtained on the path of devotion (Bhakti) as on that of knowledge. Indeed, the highest devotion (Para Bhakti) is not different from Knowledge. Both are Realization. But, whilst Liberation (Mukti) is attainable by either method, there are other marked differences between the two. A Dhyana Yogin should not neglect his body knowing that as he is both mind and matter, each reacts, the one upon the other. Neglect or mere mortification of the body is more apt to produce disordered imagination than a true spiritual experience. He is not concerned, however, with the body in the sense that the Hatha Yogin is. It is possible to be a successful Dhyana Yogin and yet to be weak in body and health, sick and short-lived.

His body, and not he himself, determines when he shall die. He cannot die at will. When he is in Samadhi, Kundalini Sakti is still sleeping in the Muladhara, and none of the physical symptoms and psychical bliss or powers (Siddhis) described as accompanying Her rousing are observed in his case. The ecstasy which he calls "Liberation while yet living" (Jivanmukti) is not a state like that of real Liberation. He may be still subject to a suffering body from which he escapes only at death, when if at all, he is liberated. His ecstasy is in the nature of a meditation which passes into the Void (Bhavana-samadhi) effected through negation of all thought-form (Chitta-Vritti) and detachment from the world—a comparatively negative process in which the positive act of raising the Central Power of the body takes no part. By his effort, the mind, which is a product of Kundalini as Prakriti Sakti, together with its worldly desires, is stilled so that the veil produced by mental functioning, is removed from Consciousness. In Laya Yoga, Kundalini Herself, when roused by the Yogin (for such rousing is his act and part), achieves for him this illumination.

But why, it may be asked, should one trouble over the body and its Central power, the more particularly as there are unusual risks and difficulties involved? The answer has been already given. There is completeness and certainty of Realization through the agency of the Power, which is Knowledge itself (Jnanarupa Sakti), an intermediate acquisition of powers (Siddhis), and intermediate and final enjoyment.

If the Ultimate Reality is the One, which exists in two aspects of quiescent enjoyment of the Self, and of liberation from all form and active enjoyment of objects, that is, as pure spirit and spirit in matter, then a complete union with Reality demands such unity in both of its aspects. It must be known both here (Iha) and there (Amutra). When rightly apprehended and practiced, there is truth in the doctrine, which teaches that man should make the best of both worlds. There is no real incompatibility between the two, provided action is taken in conformity with the universal law of manifestation. It is held to be false teaching that happiness hereafter can only be had by absence of enjoyment now, or in deliberately sought for suffering and mortification. It is the one Siva who is the Supreme Blissful Experience and who appears in the form of man with a life of mingled pleasure and pain.

Both happiness here and the bliss of Liberation here and hereafter may be attained, if the identity of these Sivas be realized in every human act. This will be achieved by making every human function, without exception, a religious act of sacrifice and worship (Yajna). In the ancient Vaidik ritual, enjoyment by way of food and drink was preceded and accompanied by ceremonial sacrifice and ritual. Such enjoyment was the fruit of the sacrifice and the gift of the Devas. At a higher stage in the life of a Sadhaka, it is offered to the One from whom all gifts come and of whom the Devatas are inferior limited forms. But this offering also involves a dualism from which the highest Monistic (Advaita) Sadhana is free. Here the individual life and the world life are known as one. And the Sadhaka, when eating or drinking or fulfilling any other of the natural functions of the body, does so, saying and feeling "Sivoham". It is not merely the separate individual who thus acts and enjoys. It is Siva who does so in and through him.

Such a one recognizes, as has been said, that his life and the play of all its activities are not a thing apart, to be held and pursued egotistically for its and his own separate sake, as though enjoyment was something to be filched from life by his own unaided strength and with a sense of separateness; but his life and all its activities are conceived as part of the Divine action in Nature (Shakti) manifesting and operating in the form of man. He realizes in the pulsating beat of his heart the rhythm, which throbs through and is the song of the Universal Life. To neglect or to deny the needs of the body, to think of it as something not divine is to neglect and deny the greater life of which it is a part, and to falsify the great doctrine of the unity of all and of the ultimate identity of Matter and Spirit. Governed by such a concept, even the lowliest physical needs take on a cosmic significance. The body is Shakti; its needs are Shakti's needs.

When man enjoys, it is Shakti who enjoys through him. In all he sees and does, it is the Mother who looks and acts; His eyes and hands are Hers. The whole body and all its functions are Her manifestations. To fully realize Her as such is to perfect this particular manifestation of Hers which is himself. Man when seeking to be the master of himself, seeks so on all the planes physical, mental and spiritual nor can they be severed, for they are all related, being but differing aspects of the one all-pervading Consciousness. Who, it may be asked, is the more divine; he who neglects and spurns the body or mind that he may attain some fancied spiritual superiority, or he who rightly cherishes both as forms of the one Spirit which they clothe?

Realization is more speedily and truly attained by discerning Spirit in and as all being and its activities, then by fleeing from and casting these aside as being either unspiritual or illusory and impediments in the path. If not rightly conceived, they may be impediments and the cause of fall; otherwise they become instruments of attainment; and what others are there to hand? And so, when acts are done in the fight feeling and frame of mind (Bhava), those acts give enjoyment; and the repeated and prolonged Bhava produces at length that divine experience (Tattva-Jnana) which is Liberation. When the Mother is seen in all things, She is at length realized as She who is beyond them all.

These general principles have their more frequent application in the life of the world before entrance on the path of Yoga proper. The Yoga here described is, however, also an application of these same principles, in so far as it is claimed that thereby both Bhukti and Mukti (enjoyment and liberation) are attained.

By the lower processes of Hatha Yoga it is sought to attain a perfect physical body, which will also be a wholly fit instrument by which the mind may function. A perfect mind, again, approaches and, in Samadhi, passes into Pure Consciousness itself. The Hatha Yogin thus seeks a body which shall be as strong as steel, healthy, free from suffering and therefore, long-lived. Master of the body he is — the master of both life and death. His lustrous form enjoys the vitality of youth. He lives as long as he has the will to live and enjoys in the world of forms. His death is the death at will (Iccha-Mrityu); when making the great and wonderfully expressive gesture of dissolution, (Samhara-Mudra) he grandly departs. But, it may be said, the Hatha Yogins do get sick and die. In the first place, the full discipline is one of difficulty and risk, and can only be pursued under the guidance of a skilled Guru. Unaided and unsuccessful practice may lead not only to disease, but death. He who seeks to conquer the Lord of death incurs the risk, on failure, of a more speedy conquest by Him.

All who attempt this Yoga do not, of course, succeed or meet with the same measure of success. Those who fail not only incur the infirmities of ordinary men, but also others brought on by practices which have been ill-pursued or for which they are not fit. Those again who do succeed, do so in varying degrees. One may prolong his life to the sacred age of 84, others to 100, others yet further. In theory at least those who are perfected (Siddhas) go from this plane when they will. All have not the same capacity or opportunity, through want of will, bodily strength, or circumstance. All may not be willing or able to follow the strict rules necessary for success. Nor does modern life offer in general the opportunities for so complete a physical culture. All men may not desire such a life or may think the attainment of it not worth the trouble involved.

Some may wish to be rid of their body and that as speedily as possible.

It is, therefore, said that it is easier to gain Liberation than Deathlessness! The former may be had by unselfishness, detachment from the world, moral and mental discipline. But to conquer death is harder than this, for these qualities and acts will not alone avail. He, who does so conquer, holds life in the hollow of one hand and, if he be a successful (Siddha) Yogin, Liberation in the other hand. He has Enjoyment and Liberation. He is the Emperor who is Master of the World and the possessor of the Bliss, which is beyond all worlds. Therefore, it is claimed by the Hatha Yogin that every Sadhana is inferior to Hatha Yoga!

The Hatha Yogin who works for Liberation does so through Laya Yoga Sadhana or Kundalini Yoga, which gives both enjoyment, and Liberation. At every center to which he rouses Kundalini he experiences special form of Bliss and gains special powers. Carrying Her to Siva of his cerebral center, he enjoys the Supreme Bliss, which in its nature is that of Liberation, and which when established in permanence is Liberation itself on the loosening of Spirit and Body.

Energy (Shakti) polarizes itself into two forms, namely, static or potential (Kundalini), and dynamic (the working forces of the body as Prana). Behind all activity there is a static background. This static center in the human body is the central Serpent Power in the Muladhara (root-support). It is the power, which is the static support (Adhara) of the whole body and all its moving Pranic forces. This Center (Kendra) of Power is a gross form of Chit or Consciousness; that is, in itself (Svarupa), it is Consciousness; and by appearance it is a Power, which, as the highest form of Force, is a manifestation of it. Just as there is a distinction (though identical at base) between the

Supreme Quiescent Consciousness and Its active Power (Shakti), so when Consciousness manifests as Energy (Sakti), it possesses the twin aspects of potential and kinetic Energy. There can be no partition in fact of Reality.

To the perfect eye of the Siddha the process of becoming is an ascription (Adhyasa). But to the imperfect eye of the Sadhaka, that is, the aspirant for Siddhi (perfected accomplishment), to the spirit which is still toiling through the lower planes and variously identifying itself with them, becoming is tending to appear and an appearance is real. The Kundalini Yoga is a rendering of Vedantic Truth from this practical point of view, and represents the world-process as a polarization in Consciousness itself. This polarity as it exists in, and as, the body is destroyed by Yoga, which disturbs the equilibrium of bodily consciousness, which consciousness is the result of the maintenance of these two poles. The human body, the potential pole of Energy which is the Supreme Power, is stirred to action, upon which the moving forces (dynamic Shakti) supported by it are drawn thereto, and the whole dynamism thus engendered moves upwards to unite with the quiescent Consciousness in the Highest Lotus.

There is polarization of Shakti into two forms—static and dynamic. In the mind or experience this polarization is patent to reflection; namely, the polarity between pure Chit and the Stress which is involved in it. This Stress or Shakti develops the mind through an infinity of forms and changes in the pure unbounded Ether of Consciousness—the Chidakasa. This analysis exhibits the primordial Shakti in the same two polar forms as before, static and dynamic. Here the polarity is most fundamental and approaches absoluteness, though of course, it is to be remembered that there is no absolute rest except in pure

Chit. Cosmic energy is in an equilibrium, which is relative and not absolute.

Passing from mind, let us take matter. The atom of modern science has ceased to be an atom in the sense of an indivisible unit of matter. According to the electron theory, the atom is a miniature universe resembling our solar system. At the center of this atomic system we have a charge of positive electricity around which a cloud of negative charges called electrons revolve. The positive charges hold each other in check so that the atom is in a condition of equilibrated energy and does not ordinarily break up, though it may do so on the dissociation which is the characteristic of all matter, but which is so clearly manifest in the radioactivity of radium. We have thus here again, a positive charge at rest at the center, and negative charges in motion round about the center. What is thus said about the atom applies to the whole cosmic system and universe. In the world-system, the planets revolve around the Sun, and that system itself is probably (taken as a whole) a moving mass around some other relatively static center, until we arrive at the Brahma-Bindu which is the point of Absolute Rest, around which all forms revolve and by which all are maintained. Similarly, in the tissues of the living body, the operative energy is polarized into two forms of energy—anabolic and catabolic, the one tending to change and the other to conserve the tissues; the actual condition of the tissues being simply the resultant of these two co-existent or concurrent activities.

In short, Shakti, when manifesting, divides itself into two polar aspects—static and dynamic — which implies that you cannot have it in a dynamic form without at the same time having it in a static form, much like the poles of a magnet. In any given sphere of activity of force, we must have, according to the cosmic principle of a static background—Shakti at rest or "coiled". This scientific truth is illustrated in the figure Kali, the Divine Mother moving as the Kinetic Shakti on the breast of Sadasiva who is the static background of pure Chit, which is actionless, the Gunamayi Mother being all activity.

The Cosmic Shakti is the collectivity (Samashti) in relation to which the Kundalini in particular bodies is the Vyashti (individual) Shakti. The body is, as I have stated, a microcosm (Kshudrabrahmanda). In the living body there is, therefore, the same polarization of which I have spoken. From the Mahakundalini the universe has sprung. In Her Supreme Form She is at rest, coiled round and one (as Chidrupini) with the Siva-bindu. She is then at rest. She next uncoils Herself to manifest. Here the three coils of which the Kundalini Yoga speaks are the three Gunas and the three and a half coil are the Prakriti and its three Gunas, together with the Vikritis. Her 50 coils are the letters of the Alphabet. As she goes on uncoiling, the Tattvas and the Matrikas, the Mother of the Varnas, issue from Her.

She is thus moving, and continues even after creation to move in the Tattvas so created. For, as they are born of movement, they continue to move. The whole world (Jagat), as the Sanskrit term implies, is moving. She thus continues creatively acting until She has evolved Prithvi, the last of the Tattvas. First She creates mind, and then matter. This latter becomes more and more dense. It has been suggested that the Mahabhutas are the Densities of modern science: Air density associated with the maximum velocity of gravity; Fire density associated with the velocity of light; Water or fluid density associated with molecular velocity and the equatorial velocity of the earth's rotation; and Earth density, that of basalt associated with the Newtonian velocity of sound. However this be, it is plain that the Bhutas represent an increasing density of matter until it reaches its three dimensional solid form. When Shakti has created this last or Prithvi Tattva, what is there further for Her to do? Nothing. She therefore then again rests. At rest, again, means that She assumes a static form. Shakti, however, is never exhausted, that is, emptied into any of its forms.

Therefore, Kundalini Shakti at this point is, as it were, the Shakti left over (though yet a plenum) after the Prithvi, the last of the Bhutas, has been created. We have thus Mahakundalini at rest as Chidrupini Shakti in the Sahasrara, the point of absolute rest; and then the body in which the relative static center is Kundalini at rest, and around this center the whole of the bodily forces move. They are Shakti, and so is Kundalini Shakti. The difference between the two is that they are Shaktis in specific differentiated forms in movement; and Kundalini Shakti is undifferentiated, residual Shakti at rest, that is, coiled.

She is coiled in the Muladhara, which means 'fundamental support', and which is at the same time the seat of the Prithvi or last solid Tattva and of the residual Shakti or Kundalini. The body may, therefore, be compared to a magnet with two poles. The Muladhara, in so far as it is the seat of Kundalini Shakti, a comparatively gross form of Chit (being Chit-Shakti and Maya Shakti), is the static pole in relation to the rest of the body, which is dynamic. The working that is the body necessarily presupposes and finds such a static support, hence the name Muladhara. In sense, the static Sakti at the Muladhara is necessarily coexistent with the creating and evolving Shakti of the body because the dynamic aspect or pole can never be without its static counterpart. In another sense, it is the residual Shakti left over after such operation.

What then happens in the accomplishment of this Yoga? Pranayama affects this static Shakti and other Yogic processes and becomes dynamic. Thus, when completely dynamic, that is when Kundalini unites with Siva in the Sahasrara, the polarization of the body gives way. The two poles are united in one and there is the state of consciousness called Samadhi. The polarization, of course, takes place in consciousness. The body actually continues to exist as an object of observation to others. It continues its organic life. But man's consciousness of his body and all other objects is withdrawn because the mind has ceased so far as his consciousness is concerned, the function having been withdrawn into its ground, which is consciousness.

How is the body sustained? In the first place, though Kundalini Sakti is the static center of the whole body as a complete conscious organism, yet each of the parts of the body and their constituent cells have their own static centers which uphold such parts or cells.

Next, the theory of the Yogins themselves is that Kundalini ascends and that the body, as a complete organism, is maintained by the nectar which flows from the union of Siva and Sakti in the Sahasrara. This nectar is an ejection of power generated by their union. The potential Kundalini Sakti becomes only partly and not wholly converted into kinetic Sakti; and yet since Sakti—even as given in the Muladhara—is an infinitude, it is not depleted; the potential store always remains unexhausted. In this case, the dynamic equivalent is a partial conversion of one mode of energy into another. If, however, the coiled power at the Muladhara became absolutely uncoiled, there would result the dissolution of the three bodies—gross, subtle and causal, and consequently, Videha-Mukti, bodiless Liberation—because the static background in relation to a particular form of existence would, according to this hypothesis, have wholly given way.

The body becomes cold as a corpse as the Sakti leaves it, not due to the depletion or privation of the static power at the Muladhara but to the concentration or convergence of the dynamic power ordinarily diffused over the whole body, so that the dynamic equivalent which is set up against the static background of Kundalini Sakti is only the diffused fivefold Prana gathered home—withdrawn from the other tissues of the body and concentrated along the axis. Thus, ordinarily, the dynamic equivalent is the Prana diffused over all the tissues: in Yoga, it is converged along the axis, the static equivalent of Kundalini Sakti enduring in both cases. Some part of the already available dynamic Prana is made to act at the base of the axis in a suitable manner, by which means the basal center or Muladhara becomes, as it were, oversaturated and reacts on the whole diffused dynamic power (or Prana) of the body by withdrawing it from the tissues and converging it along the line of the axis.

In this way, the diffused dynamic equivalent becomes the converged dynamic equivalent along the axis. What, according to this view, ascends is not the whole Sakti but an eject like condensed lightning, which at length reaches the Parama-Sivasthana. There the Central Power, which upholds the individual world-Consciousness, is merged in the Supreme Consciousness. The limited consciousness, transcending the passing concepts of worldly life, directly intuits the unchanging Reality which underlies the whole phenomenal flow. When Kundalini Sakti sleeps in the Muladhara, man is awake to the world; when she awakes to unite, and does unite, with the supreme static Consciousness which is Siva, then consciousness is asleep to the world and is one with the Light of all things.

The main principle is that when awakened, Kundalini Sakti, either Herself or Her eject, ceases to be a static Power which sustains the world-consciousness, the content of which is held only so long as She sleeps; and when once set in movement is drawn to that other static center in the Thousand-petaled Lotus (Sahasrara) which is Herself in union with the Siva-consciousness or the consciousness of ecstasy beyond the world of form. When Kundalini sleeps, man is awake to this world. When She wakes, he sleeps— that is, loses all consciousness of the world and enters his causal body. In Yoga, he passes beyond to formless Consciousness.

Glory, glory to Mother Kundalini, who through Her Infinite Grace and Power, kindly leads the Sadhaka from Chakra to Chakra and illumines his intellect and makes him realize his identity with the Supreme Brahman! May Her blessings be upon you all!

THE FOUR STAGES OF SOUND

The Vedas form the sound-manifestation of Ishvara. That sound has four divisions, — Para which finds manifestation only in Prana, Pasyanti which finds manifestation in the mind, Madhyama which finds manifestation in the Indriyas, and Vaikhari which finds manifestation in articulate expression.

Articulation is the last and grossest expression of divine sound-energy. The highest manifestation of sound-energy, the primal voice, the divine voice is Para. The Para voice becomes the root-ideas or germ-thoughts. It is the first manifestation of voice. In Para the sound remains in an undifferentiated form. Para, Pasyanti, Madhyama and Vaikhari are the various gradations of sound. Madhyama is the intermediate unexpressed state of sound. Its seat is the heart.

The seat of Pasyanti is the navel or the Manipura Chakra. Yogins who have subtle inner vision can experience the Pasyanti state of a word which has color and form, which is common for all languages and which has the vibrating homogeneity of sound. Indians, Europeans, Americans, Africans, Japanese, birds, and beasts — all experience the same Bhavana of a thing in the Pasyanti state of voice or sound. Gesture is a sort of mute subtle language. It is one and the same for all persons. Any individual of any country will make the same gesture by holding his hand to his mouth in a particular manner, when he is thirsty. As one and the same power or Shakti working through the ears becomes hearing, through the eyes becomes seeing and so forth, the same Pasyanti assumes different forms of sound when materialized. The Lord manifests Himself through his Mayaic power first as Para Vani in the Muladhara Chakra at the navel, then as Madhyama in the heart and then eventually as Vaikhari in the throat and mouth. This is the divine descent of His voice. All the Vaikhari is His voice only. It is the voice of the Virat Purusha.

STOTRAS
(Prayer or Hymns)

GURU STOTRA

"Salutations to the Guru who has made it possible to realize Him by whom all this world, animate and inanimate, movable and immovable, is pervaded."

"Salutations to Omkara, which gives whatever one desires and also liberation to those who meditate always on Omkara that is united with the Bindu."

"Salutations to the Guru who is established in Knowledge and Power, who is adorned with the garland of Knowledge and who grants both worldly prosperity and liberation."

DEVI STOTRA

"I seek refuge in Tripurasundari, the wife of the three-eyed One, who lives in the Kadamba forest, who is seated on the golden disc and dwells in the six lotuses of the Yogins, ever flashing like lightning in the heart of the perfected ones, whose beauty excels that of the Japa flower and whose forehead is adorned by the full-moon."

"O Thou Self of everything, of whatever thing existing at whatever place or time, whether cause or effect, Thou art the Power behind that; how canst Thou be praised?"

"Thou art the Supreme Knowledge, Maya, intellect, memory, delusion and the great Prowess of the gods as well as of the demons."

SIVA STOTRA

"Sins committed in action—with the hands and feet or by speech, or by the body, or by the ears and eyes, — or by those done in thoughts, — forgive all these sins whether of commission or omission. Glory be unto Thee, Thou ocean of mercy! Glory be unto Thee O Mahadeva, O Shambho!"
—*Sri Sankaracharya*

TO THE KUNDALINI — THE MOTHER OF THE UNIVERSE

"What Yogis now, what Rishis of old,
The greatness of that Mother hath told,
Who from her own breast gave birth To
the sky and to the earth.

Thou hung the Heavens in empty space,
And holds the earth in its place,
Thou made and lighted up the sun
To stay and shine this earth upon.

Thy power transcendent, since their birth
Asunder holds the heaven and earth,
As chariot wheels are kept apart
By axles made thru workman's art.

In Shakti, who with thee can vie,
Thou fills the earth, the air, the sky;
Thy presence, unperceived, extends
Beyond the world's remotest ends.

A million earths, if such there be,
A million skies fall short of thee;
A billion suns can not out shine
The effulgence of thy light divine.

The worlds, which mortals boundless deem
To thee but as a handful seem.
Mother, Thou art without a peer.
On earth, or in yonder heavenly sphere.

Thee, God, such matchless powers adorn
That thou without a foe was born.
Thou art the Lord of Lords,
Adored by Men — revered by Gods.

The circling times which wear away,
All else, to thee can not decay;
Thou shinest on in youthful force,
While countless Yugas run their course.

Unvexed by cares, or fears, or strife,
In bliss serene flow on thy life,
With faith we claim thine aid divine,
As thou art Mother, and we are thine.

Metrical translation from the Sanskrit writers, by Mr. J. Muir, with modifications by Rishi Singh Gherwal

Chapter Two

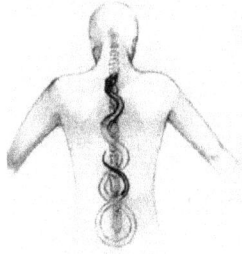

COSMIC ENERGY

O Divine Mother Kundalini, the Divine Cosmic Energy that is hidden in men! Thou art Kali, Durga, Adisakti, Rajarajeswari, Tripurasundari, Maha-Lakshmi, Maha-Sarasvati! Thou hast put on all these names and forms. Thou hast manifested as Prana, electricity, force, magnetism, cohesion, and gravitation in this universe. This whole universe rests in Thy bosom. Crores of salutations unto thee. O Mother of this world! Lead me on to open the Sushumna Nadi and take Thee along the Chakras to Sahasrara Chakra and to merge myself in Thee and Thy consort, Lord Siva.

Kundalini Yoga is that Yoga which treats of Kundalini Sakti, the six centers of spiritual energy (Shat Chakras), the arousing of the sleeping Kundalini Sakti and its union with Lord Siva in Sahasrara Chakra, at the crown of the head. This is an exact science. This is also known as Laya Yoga. The six centers are pierced (Chakra Bheda) by the passing of Kundalini Sakti to the top of the head. 'Kundala' means 'coiled'. Her form is like a coiled serpent. Hence the name Kundalini.

All agree that the one aim which man has in all his acts is to secure happiness for himself. The highest as well as the ultimate end of man must, therefore, be to attain eternal, infinite, unbroken, supreme happiness. This happiness can be had in one's own Self or Atman only. Therefore, search within to attain this eternal Bliss.

The thinking faculty is present only in human being. Man only can reason, reflect and exercise judgment. It is man only who can compare and contrast, who can think of pros and cons and who can draw inferences and conclusions. This is the reason why he alone is able to attain God-consciousness. That man who simply eats and drinks and who does not exercise his mental faculty in Self-realization is only a brute.

O worldly-minded persons! Wake up from the sleep of Ajnana. Open your eyes. Stand up to acquire knowledge of Atman. Do spiritual Sadhana, awaken the Kundalini Sakti and get that 'sleepless-sleep' (Samadhi). Drown yourself in Atman.

Chitta is the mental substance. It takes various forms. These forms constitute Vrittis. It gets transformed (Parinama). These transformations or modifications are the thought-waves, whirlpools or Vrittis. If the Chitta thinks of a mango, the Vritti of a mango is formed in the lake of Chitta. This will subside and another Vritti will be formed when it thinks of milk. Countless Vrittis are rising and subsiding in the ocean of Chitta. These Vrittis cause restlessness of mind. Why do Vrittis arise from the Chitta? Because of Samskaras and Vasanas. If you annihilate all Vasanas, all Vrittis will subside by themselves.

When a Vritti subsides it leaves a definite impression in the subconscious mind. It is known as Samskara or latent impression. The sum total of all Samskaras is known as "Karmasaya" or receptacle of works. This is called Sanchita

Karma (accumulated works). When a man leaves the physical body, he carries with him his astral body of 17 Tattvas and the Karmasaya as well, to the mental plane. This Karmasaya is burnt by highest knowledge obtained through Asamprajnata Samadhi.

During concentration you will have to collect carefully the dissipated rays of the mind. Vrittis will be ever-rising from the ocean of Chitta. You will have to put down the waves as they arise. If all the waves subside, the mind becomes calm and serene. Then the Yogi enjoys peace and bliss. Therefore real happiness is within. You will have to get it through control of mind and not through money, women, children, name, fame, rank or power.

Purity of mind leads to perfection in Yoga. Regulate your conduct when you deal with others. Have no feeling of jealousy towards others. Be compassionate. Do not hate sinners. Be kind to all. Develop complacency towards superiors. Success in Yoga will be rapid if you put in your maximum energy in your Yogic practice. You must have a keen longing for liberation and intense Vairagya also. You must be sincere and earnest. Intent and constant meditation is necessary for entering into Samadhi.

He who has firm faith in Srutis and Shastras, who has Sadachara (right conduct), who constantly engages himself in the service of his Guru and who is free from lust, anger, Moha, greed and vanity easily crosses this ocean of Samsara and attains Samadhi quickly. Just as fire burns a heap of dried leaves, so also the fire of Yoga burns all Karmas. The Yogi attains Kaivalya. Through Samadhi, the Yogi gets intuition. Real knowledge flashes in him within a second.

Neti, Dhauti, Basti, Nauli, Asanas, Mudras, etc., keep the body healthy and strong, and under perfect control. But they are not the be-all and end-all of Yoga. These Kriyas will help you in your practice of Dhyana. Dhyana will culminate in Samadhi, Self-realization. He who practices Hatha Yogic Kriyas is not a Purna Yogi. He who has entered into Asamprajnata Samadhi only is a Purna Yogi. He is a Svatantra Yogi (absolutely independent).

Samadhi is of two kinds, viz., Jada Samadhi and Chaitanya Samadhi. A Hatha Yogi through the practice of Khechari Mudra can shut himself up in a box and remain underneath the ground for months and years. There is no higher supernatural knowledge in this kind of Samadhi. This is Jada Samadhi. In Chaitanya Samadhi, there is perfect 'awareness'. The Yogi comes down with new, super-sensuous wisdom.

When a man practices Yogic Kriyas, naturally various kinds of Siddhis are acquired. The Siddhis are hindrances to Realization. The Yogi should not at all care for these Siddhis, if he wants to advance further and get the highest realization, the final Goal. He who runs after Siddhis will become the biggest householder and a worldly-minded man. Self-realization only is the Goal. The sum total of knowledge of this universe is nothing when compared to the spiritual knowledge that is obtained through Self-realization.

Ascend the path of Yoga cautiously. Remove the weeds, thorns and the sharp angular pebbles on the way. Name and fame are the angular pebbles. Subtle under-current of lust is the weed. Attachment to family, children, money, disciples, Chelas or Ashram is the thorn. These are forms of Maya. They do not allow the aspirants to march further. They serve as the stumbling blocks. The aspirant gets false Tushti, stops his Sadhana, imagines foolishly that he has realized, and tries to elevate others. This is like a blind man leading the blind. When the Yogic student starts an Ashram, slowly luxury creeps in. The original Vairagya gradually wanes. He loses what he has gained and is unconscious of his downfall. Ashram develops begging mentality and institutional egoism. He is the same householder now in some other form (Rupantara-bheda) though he is in the garb of a Sannyasin. O aspirants, beware! I warn you seriously. Never build Ashrams. Remember the watchwords: "SECLUSION, MEDITATION, DEVOTION." March direct to the goal. Never give up the Sadhana zeal and Vairagya until you realize Bhuma, the highest goal. Do not entangle yourself in the wheel of name, fame and Siddhis.

Nirvikalpa is the state of superconsciousness. There are no Vikalpas of any sort in this condition. This is the Goal of life. All the mental activities cease now. The functions of the intellect and ten Indriyas cease entirely. The aspirant rests now in Atman. There is no distinction between subject and object. The world and the pairs of opposites vanish completely. This is a state beyond all relativity. The aspirant gets knowledge of Self, supreme peace and infinite, indescribable bliss. This is also called Yogaroodha state.

When Kundalini is taken to the Sahasrara and when it is united with Lord Siva, perfect Samadhi ensues. The Yogic student drinks the Nectar of Immortality. He has reached the Goal. Mother Kundalini has done Her task now. Glory to Mother Kundalini! May Her blessings be upon you all!
Om Shantih! Shantih! Shantih!

OM

EXPERIENCES ON AWAKENING OF KUNDALINI

During meditation you behold divine visions, experience divine smell, divine taste, divine touch, hear divine Anahata sounds. You receive instructions from God. These indicate that the Kundalini Shakti has been awakened. When there is throbbing in Muladhara, when hairs stand on their roots, when Uddiyana, Jalandhara and Mulabandha come involuntarily, know that Kundalini has awakened.

When the breath stops without any effort, when Kevala Kumbhaka comes by itself without any exertion, know that Kundalini Shakti has become active. When you feel currents of Prana rising up to the Sahasrara, when you experience bliss, when you repeat Om automatically, when there are no thoughts of the world in the mind, know that Kundalini Shakti has awakened.

When, in your meditation, the eyes become fixed on Trikuti, the middle of the eyebrows, when the Shambhavi Mudra operates, know that Kundalini has become active. When you feel vibrations of Prana in different parts inside your body, when you experience jerks like the shocks of electricity, know that Kundalini has become active. During meditation when you feel as if there is no body, when your eyelids become closed and do not open in spite of your exertion, when electric-like currents flow up and down the nerves, know that Kundalini has awakened.

When you meditate, when you get inspiration and insight, when the nature unfolds its secrets to you, all doubts disappear, you understand clearly the meaning of the Vedic texts, know that Kundalini has become active. When your body becomes light like air, when you have a balanced mind in perturbed condition, when you possess inexhaustible energy for work, know that Kundalini has become active.

When you get divine intoxication, when you develop power of oration, know that Kundalini has awakened. When you involuntarily perform different Asanas or poses of Yoga without the least pain or fatigue, know that Kundalini has become active. When you compose beautiful sublime hymns and poetry involuntarily, know that Kundalini has become active.

THE GRADATIONAL ASCENT OF THE MIND

The Chakras are centers of Shakti as vital force. In other words, these are centers of Pranashakti manifested by Pranavayu in the living body, the presiding Devatas of which are the names for the Universal Consciousness as It manifests in the form of these centers. The Chakras are not perceptible to the gross senses. Even if they were perceptible in the living body which they help to organize, they disappear with the disintegration of organism at death.

Purity of mind leads to perfection in Yoga. Regulate your conduct when you deal with others. Have no feeling of jealousy towards others. Be compassionate. Do not hate sinners. Be kind to all. Success in Yoga will be rapid if you put your maximum energy in your Yogic practice. You must have a keen longing for liberation and intense Vairagya also. You must be sincere and earnest. Intense and constant meditation is necessary for entering into Samadhi. The mind of a worldly man with base desires and passions moves in the Muladhara and Svadhishthana Chakras or centers situated near the anus and the reproductive organ respectively.

If one's mind becomes purified the mind rises to the Manipura Chakra or the center in the navel and experiences some power and joy.

If the mind becomes more purified, it rises to the Anahata Chakra or center in the heart, experiences bliss and visualizes the effulgent form of the Ishta Devata or the tutelary deity.

When the mind gets highly purified, when meditation and devotion become intense and profound the mind rises to Visuddha Chakra or the center in the throat, and experiences more and more powers and bliss. Even when the mind has reached this center, there is a possibility for it to come down to the lower centers.

When the Yogi reaches the Ajna Chakra or the center between the two eyebrows he attains Samadhi and realizes the Supreme Self, or Brahman. There is a slight sense of separateness between the devotee and Brahman.

If he reaches the spiritual center in the brain, the Sahasrara Chakra, the thousand-petaled lotus, the Yogi attains Nirvikalpa Samadhi or superconscious state. He becomes one with the non-dual Brahman. All sense of separateness dissolves. This is the highest plane of consciousness or supreme Asamprajnata Samadhi. Kundalini unites with Siva.

The Yogi may come down to the center in the throat to give instructions to the students and do good to others (Lokasamgraha).

PRANAYAMA FOR AWAKENING KUNDALINI

When you practice the following, concentrate on the Muladhara Chakra at the base of the spinal column, which is triangular in form and which is the seat of the Kundalini Shakti. Close the right nostril with your right thumb. Inhale through the left nostril till you count 3 Oms slowly. Imagine that you are drawing the Prana with the atmospheric air. Then close the left nostril with your little and ring fingers of the right hand. Then retain the breath for 12 Oms. Send the current down the spinal column straight into the triangular lotus, the Muladhara Chakra. Imagine that the nerve-current is striking against the lotus and awakening the Kundalini. Then slowly exhale through the right nostril counting 6 Oms. Repeat the process from the right nostril as stated above, using the same units, and having the same imagination and feeling. This Pranayama will awaken the Kundalini quickly. Do it 3 times in the morning and 3 times in the evening. Increase the number and time gradually and cautiously according to your strength and capacity. In this Pranayama, concentration on the Muladhara Chakra is the important thing. Kundalini will be awakened quickly if the degree of concentration is intense and if the Pranayama is practiced regularly.

KUNDALINI PRANAYAMA

In this Pranayama, the Bhavana is more important than the ratio between Puraka, Kumbhaka and Rechaka. Sit in Padma or Siddha Asana, facing the East or the North. After mentally prostrating to the lotus-feet of the Sat-guru and reciting Stotras in praise of God and Guru, commence doing this Pranayama which will easily lead to the awakening of the Kundalini.

Inhale deeply, without making any sound. As you inhale, feel that the Kundalini lying dormant in the Muladhara Chakra is awakened and is going up from Chakra to Chakra. At the conclusion of the Puraka, have the Bhavana that the Kundalini has reached the Sahasrara. The more vivid the visualization of Chakra after Chakra, the more rapid will be your progress in this Sadhana.

Retain the breath for a short while. Repeat the Pranava or your Ishta Mantra. Concentrate on the Sahasrara Chakra. Feel that the Grace of Mother Kundalini has dispelled the darkness of ignorance enveloping your soul. Feel that your whole being is pervaded by light, power and wisdom.

Slowly exhale now. And, as you exhale feel that the Kundalini Shakti is gradually descending from the Sahasrara, and from Chakra to Chakra, to the Muladhara Chakra.

Now begin the process again. It is impossible to extol this wonderful Pranayama adequately. It is the magic wand for attaining perfection very quickly. Even a few days' practice will convince you of its remarkable glory. Start from today, this very moment.

May God bless you with joy, bliss and immortality.

KUNDALINI

The word Kundalini is a familiar one to all students of Yoga, as it is well known as the power, in the form of a coiled serpent, residing in Muladhara Chakra, the first of the seven Chakras, the other six being Svadhishthana,

Manipuraka, Anahata, Visuddha, Ajna and Sahasrara, in order.

All Sadhanas in the form of Japa, meditation, Kirtan and prayer as well as all development of virtues, and observance of austerities like truth, non-violence and continence are at best calculated only to awaken this serpent-power and make it to pass through all the succeeding Chakras beginning from Svadhishthana to Sahasrara, the latter otherwise called as the thousand-petaled lotus, the seat of Sadasiva or the Parabrahman or the Absolute separated from whom the Kundalini or the Shakti lies at the Muladhara, and to unite with whom the Kundalini passes through all the Chakras, as explained above, conferring liberation on the aspirant who assiduously practices Yoga or the technique of uniting her with her Lord and gets success also in his effort.

In worldly-minded people, given to enjoyment of sensual and sexual pleasures, this Kundalini power is sleeping because of the absence of any stimulus in the form of spiritual practices, as the power generated through such practices alone awakens that serpent-power, and not any other power derived through the possession of worldly riches and affluence. When the aspirant seriously practices all the disciplines as enjoined in the Shastras, and as instructed by the preceptor, in whom the Kundalini would have already been awakened and reached its abode or Sadasiva, acquiring which blessed achievement alone a person becomes entitled to act as a Guru or spiritual preceptor, guiding and helping others also to achieve the same end, the veils or layers enmeshing Kundalini begin to be cleared and finally are torn asunder and the serpent-power is pushed or driven, as it were upwards.

Supersensual visions appear before the mental eye of the aspirant, new worlds with indescribable wonders and charms unfold themselves before the Yogi, planes after planes reveal their existence and grandeur to the practitioner and the Yogi gets divine knowledge, power and bliss, in increasing degrees, when Kundalini passes through Chakra after Chakra, making them to bloom in all their glory which before the touch of Kundalini, do not give out their powers, emanating their divine light and fragrance and reveal the divine secrets and phenomena, which lie concealed from the eyes of worldly-minded people who would refuse to believe of their existence even.

When the Kundalini ascends one Chakra or Yogic center, the Yogi also ascends one step or rung upward in the Yogic ladder; one more page, the next page, he reads in the divine book; the more the Kundalini travels upwards, the Yogi also advances towards the goal or spiritual perfection in relation to it. When the Kundalini reaches the sixth center or the Ajna Chakra, the Yogi gets the vision of Personal God or Saguna Brahman, and when the serpent-power reaches the last, the top center, or Sahasrara Chakra, or the Thousand-petaled lotus, the Yogi loses his individuality in the ocean of Sat-Chit-Ananda or the Existence-Knowledge-Bliss Absolute and becomes one with the Lord or Supreme Soul. He is no longer an ordinary man, not even a simple Yogi, but a fully illumined sage, having conquered the eternal and unlimited divine kingdom, a hero having won the battle against illusion, a Mukta or liberated one having crossed the ocean of ignorance or the transmigratory existence, and a superman having the authority and capacity to save the other struggling souls of the relative world. Scriptures hail him most, in the maximum possible glorifying way, and his achievement. Celestial beings envy him, not excluding the Trinity even, viz., Brahma, Vishnu and Siva.

Kundalini And Tantrik Sadhana

Kundalini Yoga actually belongs to Tantrik Sadhana, which gives a detailed description about this serpent-power and the Chakras, as mentioned above. Mother Divine, the active aspect of the Existence-Knowledge-Bliss Absolute, resides in the body of men and women in the form of Kundalini, and the entire Tantrik Sadhana aims at awakening Her, and making Her to unite with the Lord, Sadasiva, in the Sahasrara, as described in the beginning in detail. Methods adopted to achieve this end in Tantrik Sadhana are Japa of the name of the Mother, prayer and various rituals.

Kundalini And Hatha Yoga

Hatha Yoga also builds up its philosophy around this Kundalini and the methods adopted in it are different from Tantrik Sadhana. Hatha Yoga seeks to awaken this Kundalini through the discipline of the physical body, purification of Nadis and controlling the Prana. Through a number of physical poses called Yoga Asanas it tones up the entire nervous system, and brings it under the conscious control of the Yogi, through Bandhas and Mudras it controls the Prana, regulates its movements and even blocks and seals it without allowing it to move, through Kriyas it purifies the inner organs of physical body and, finally, through Pranayama it brings the mind itself under the control of the Yogi. Kundalini is made to go upwards towards Sahasrara through these combined methods.

Kundalini And Raja Yoga

But Raja Yoga mentions nothing about this Kundalini, but propounds a still subtle, higher path, philosophical and rational, and asks the aspirant to control the mind, to withdraw all the senses and to plunge in meditation. Unlike Hatha Yoga which is mechanical and mystical, Raja Yoga teaches a technique with eight limbs, appealing to the heart and intellect of aspirants. It advocates moral and ethical development through its Yama and Niyama, helps the intellectual and cultural development through Svadhyaya or study of holy Scriptures, satisfies the emotional and devotional aspect of human nature by enjoining to surrender oneself to the will of the Creator, has an element of mysticism by including Pranayama also as one of the eight limbs and finally, prepares the aspirant for unbroken meditation on the Absolute through a penultimate step of concentration. Neither in philosophy nor in its prescription of methods of Raja Yoga mentions about Kundalini, but sets the human mind and Chitta as its targets to be destroyed as they alone make the individual soul to forget its real nature and brings on it birth and death and all the woes of phenomenal existence.

Kundalini And Vedanta

But when we come to Vedanta, there is no question about Kundalini or any type of mystical and mechanical methods. It is all enquiry and philosophical speculation. According to Vedanta the only thing to be destroyed is ignorance about one's real nature, and this ignorance cannot be destroyed either by study, or by Pranayama, or by work, or by any amount of physical twisting and torturing, but only by knowing one's real nature, which is Sat-Chit-Ananda or Existence-Knowledge-Bliss. Man is divine, free and one with the Supreme Spirit always, which he forgets and identifies himself with matter, which itself is an illusory appearance and a superimposition on the spirit. Liberation is freedom from ignorance and the aspirant is advised to constantly dissociate himself from all limitations and identify himself with the all-pervading, non-dual, blissful, peaceful, homogeneous spirit or Brahman. When meditation becomes intensified, in the ocean of Existence or rather the individuality is blotted or blown out completely. Just as a drop of water let on a frying pan is immediately sucked and vanishes from cognition, the individual consciousness is sucked in by the Universal Consciousness and is absorbed in it. According to Vedanta there cannot be real liberation in a state of multiplicity, and the state of complete Oneness is the goal to be aspired for, towards which alone the entire creation is slowly moving on.

Chapter Three

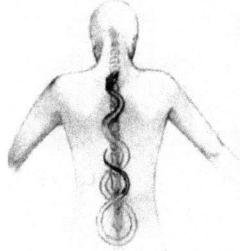

THE FOUNDATION

Patanjali-vyasamukhan gurunanyamscha bhaktitah; Natosmi vangmanah-kayairajnanadhvanta-bhaskaran—We offer our obeisance by word, mind and body to Patanjali, Vyasa and to all other Rishis and Yogic Masters who are like so many Suns to remove the darkness of Ajnana (ignorance).

Foundation—Vairagya

Man, ignorant of his true Divine nature, vainly tries to secure happiness in the perishable objects of this illusory sense-universe. Every man in this world is restless, discontented and dissatisfied. He feels actually that he is in want of something, the nature of which he does not really understand. He seeks the rest and peace that he feels he is in need of, in the accomplishment of ambitious projects. But he finds that worldly greatness when secured is a delusion and a snare. He doubtless does not find any happiness in it. He gets degrees, diplomas, titles, honors, powers, name and fame; he marries; he begets children; in short, he gets all that he imagines would give him happiness. But yet, he finds no rest and peace.

Are you not ashamed to repeat the same process of eating, sleeping and talking again and again? Are you not really fed up with the illusory objects created by the jugglery of Maya? Have you got a single sincere friend in this universe? Is there any difference between an animal and the so-called dignified human being with boasted intellect, if he does not do any spiritual Sadhana daily, for Self-realization? How long do you want to remain a slave of passion, Indriyas, woman and body? Fie on those miserable wretches who revel in filth and who have forgotten their real Atmic nature and their hidden powers!

The so-called educated persons are refined sensualists only. Sensual pleasure is no pleasure at all. Indriyas are deceiving you at every moment. Pleasure mixed with pain, sorrow, fear, sin, and diseases is no pleasure at all. The happiness that depends upon perishable objects is no happiness. If your wife dies, you weep. If you lose money or property, you are drowned in sorrow. How long do you want to remain in that abject, degraded state? Those who waste their precious life in eating, sleeping and chatting without doing any Sadhana are brutes only.

You have forgotten your real Svarupa or purpose of life on account of Avidya, Maya, Moha and Raga. The two currents of Raga and Dvesha toss you up hither and thither aimlessly. You are caught up in Samsara-Chakra on account of your egoism, Vasanas, Trishnas and passions of various sorts. You want a *Nitya* (eternal), *Nirupadhika* (independent), *Niratisaya* (Infi nite) *Ananda*. This you will find in your realization of the Self only. Then alone will all your miseries and tribulations melt away. You have taken this body only to achieve this end. *"Din nike bite jate hain—* The days are passing away quickly."* The day has come and gone. Will you waste the night also?

"Aashaya badhyate loko karmana bahu-chintaya; Ayukshinam na janati tasmat jagrata jagrata — You are bound in this world by desires, actions and manifold anxieties. Therefore you do not know that your life is slowly decaying and is wasted. Therefore wake up, wake up."
Now wake up. Open your eyes. Apply diligently to spiritual Sadhana. Never waste even a minute. Many Yogins and Jnanins, Dattatreya, Patanjali, Christ, Buddha, Gorakhnath, Matsyendranath, Ram Das and others have already trodden the spiritual path and realized through Sadhana. Follow their teachings and instructions implicitly.

Courage, Power, Strength, Wisdom, Joy and Happiness are your Divine heritage, your birth-right. Get them all through proper Sadhana. It will be simply preposterous to think that your Guru will do the Sadhana for you. You are your own redeemer. Gurus and Acharyas will show you the spiritual path, remove doubts and troubles and give some inspiration. You will have to tread the Spiritual Path. Remember this point well. You will have to place each step yourself in the Spiritual Path. Therefore do real Sadhana. Free yourself from death and birth and enjoy the Highest Bliss.

What Is Yoga?
The word 'Yoga' comes from a Sanskrit root 'Yuj' which means to join. In its spiritual sense it is that process by which the identity of the Jivatma and Paramatma is realized by the Yogins. The human soul is brought into conscious communion with God. Yoga is restraining the mental modifications. Yoga is that inhibition of the functions of the mind which leads to abidance of the spirit in his real nature. The inhibition of these functions of the mind is by Abhyasa and Vairagya" (Yoga Sutras).

Yoga is the Science that teaches the method of joining the human spirit with God. Yoga is the Divine Science which disentangles the Jiva from the phenomenal world of sense-objects and links him with the *Ananta Ananda* (Infinite Bliss), *Parama Shanti* (Supreme Peace), joy of an Akhanda character and Power that are inherent attributes of the Absolute. Yoga gives Mukti through Asamprajnata Samadhi by destroying all the Sankalpas of all antecedent mental functions. No Samadhi is possible without awakening the Kundalini. When the Yogi attains the highest stage, all his Karmas are burnt and he gets liberation from Samsara-Chakra.

The Importance Of Kundalini Yoga

In Kundalini Yoga the creating and sustaining Sakti of the whole body is actually and truly united with Lord Siva. The Yogi goads Her to introduce him to Her Lord. The rousing of Kundalini Sakti and Her Union with Lord Siva effects the state of *Samadhi* (Ecstatic union) and spiritual *Anubhava* (experience). It is She who gives Knowledge or Jnana, for She is Herself That. Kundalini Herself, when awakened by the Yogins, achieves for them the Jnana (illumination).

Kundalini can be awakened by various means and these different methods are called by different names, viz., Raja Yoga, Hatha Yoga, etc. The practitioner of this Kundalini Yoga claims, that it is higher than any other process and that Samadhi attained thereby is more perfect. The reason that they allege, is this: —In Dhyana Yoga, ecstasy takes place through detachment from the world and mental concentration leading the variety of mental operation (*Vritti*) of the uprising of pure consciousness unhindered by the limitations of the mind. The degree to which this unveiling of consciousness is effected, depends upon the meditative power, Dhyana Sakti, of the Sadhaka and the extent of detachment from the world. On the other hand, Kundalini is all Sakti and is therefore Jnana Sakti Herself—bestows Jnana and Mukti, when awakened by the Yogins. Secondly, in Kundalini Yoga there is not merely a Samadhi through meditation, but the central power of the Jiva, carries with it the forms of both body and mind. The union in that sense is claimed to be more complete than that enacted through methods only. Though in both cases the body-consciousness is lost, in Kundalini Yoga not only the mind but the body also, in so far as it is represented by its central power, is actually united with Lord Siva at the Sahasrara Chakra. This union (Samadhi) produces *Bhukti* (enjoyment) which a Dhyana Yogi does not possess. A Kundalini Yogi has both *Bhukti* (enjoyment) and *Mukti* (liberation) in the fullest and literal sense. Hence this Yoga is claimed to be the foremost of all Yogas. When the sleeping Kundalini is awakened by Yogic Kriyas, it forces a passage upwards through the different Chakras (Shat-Chakra *Bheda*). It excites or stimulates them into intense activity. During its ascent, layer after layer of the mind becomes fully opened. All *Kleshas* (afflictions) and the three kinds of Taapa will vanish. The Yogi experiences various visions, powers, bliss and knowledge. When it reaches Sahasrara Chakra in the brain, the Yogi gets the maximum knowledge, Bliss, power and Siddhis. He reaches the highest rung in the Yogic ladder. He gets perfectly detached from body and mind. He becomes free in all respects. He is a full-blown Yogi (*Purna Yogi*).

Important Qualifications Of A Sadhaka

When the whole vitality is sapped from the body one cannot do any rigid Sadhana. Youth is the best period for Yoga Abhyasa. This is the first and the foremost qualification of a Sadhaka; there must be vigor and vitality. One who has a calm mind, who has faith in the words of his Guru and Sastras, who is moderate in eating and sleeping and who has the intense longing for deliverance from the Samsara-Chakra is a qualified person for the practice of Yoga.

"*Ahamkaram balam darpam kamam krodham parigraham; Vimuchya nirmamah santo brahmabhuyaya kalpate* - Having cast aside egoism, violence, arrogance, desire, wrath, covetousness, selfless and peaceful—he is fit to become ETERNAL."

Those who are addicted to sensual pleasures or those who are arrogant and proud, dishonest, untruthful, diplomatic, cunning and treacherous and who disrespect the Guru, Sadhus and elders and take pleasure in vain controversies and worldly actions, can never attain success in Yogic practices.

Kama, Krodha, Lobha, Moha, Mada, and all other impurities should be completely annihilated. One cannot become pure and perfect when one has so many impure qualities.

Sadhakas should develop the following virtuous qualities:

Straightforwardness, service to Guru, the sick and old persons, Ahimsa, Brahmacharya, spontaneous generosity, Titiksha, Sama Drishti, Samata, spirit of service, selflessness, tolerance, Mitahara, humility, honesty and other virtues to an enormous degree. Aspirants will not at all be benefited in any way in the absence of these virtues even if they exert much to awaken the Kundalini through Yogic exercises.

Aspirants should freely open their hearts to their Guru. They must be frank and candid. They should give up the self-assertive, Rajasic vehemence, vanity and arrogance, and carry out their master's instructions with Sraddha and Prem. Constant self-justification is a dangerous habit for a Sadhaka.

Energy is wasted in too much talking, unnecessary worry and vain fear. Gossiping and tall-talk should be given up entirely. A real Sadhaka is a man of few words, to the point and that too on spiritual matters only. Sadhakas should always remain alone. Mouna is a great *desideratum*. Mixing with householders is highly dangerous for a Sadhaka. The company of a householder is far more injurious than the company of a woman. Mind has the power to imitate.

Yogic Diet

A Sadhaka should observe perfect discipline. He must be civil, polite, courteous, gentle, noble and gracious in his behavior. He must have perseverance, adamantine will, asinine patience and *leech-like tenacity* in Sadhana. He must be perfectly self-controlled, pure and devoted to the Guru.

A glutton or one who is a slave of his senses with several bad habits, is unfit for the spiritual path.

"Mitaharam vina yastu yogarambham tu karayet; Nanarogo bhavettasya kinchit yogo na siddhyati "Without observing moderation of diet, if one takes to the Yogic practices, he cannot obtain any benefit but gets various diseases" (Ghe. Sam. V-16).

Food plays a prominent place in Yoga-Sadhana. An aspirant should be very careful in the selection of articles of Sattvic nature especially in the beginning of his Sadhana period. Later on when Siddhi is attained, drastic dietetic restrictions can be removed.

Purity of food leads to purity of mind. Sattvic food helps meditation. The discipline of food is very necessary for Yogic Sadhana. If the tongue is controlled, all the other Indriyas are controlled.

"Ahara-suddhau sattva-suddhih, sattva-suddhau dhruva smritih; Smriti-lambhe sarva-granthinam viprarnokshah—By the purity of food follows the purification of the inner nature, by the purification of the nature, memory becomes firm and on strengthening the memory, follows the loosening of all ties and the wise get Moksha thereby."

Sattvic Articles

I will give you a list of Sattvic articles for a Sadhaka. Milk, red rice, barley, wheat, *Havishannam*, *Charu*, cream, cheese, butter, green dal (*Moong dal*), Badam (almonds), *Misri* (sugar-candy), *Kismis*(raisins), *Kichidi*, *Pancha Shakha* vegetables (*Seendil, Chakravarty, Ponnan gani, Chirukeerai* and *Vellaicharnai*), *Lowki* vegetable, plantain-stem, *Parwal*, *Bhindi* (lady's finger), pomegranates, sweet oranges, grapes, apples, bananas, mangoes, dates, honey, dried ginger, black pepper, etc., are the Sattvic articles of diet prescribed for the Yoga Abhyasis.

Charu: Boil half a seer of milk along with some boiled rice, ghee and sugar. This is an excellent food for Yogins. This is for the daytime. For the night, half a seer of milk will do.

Milk should not be too much boiled. It should be removed from the fire as soon as the boiling point is reached. Too much boiling destroys the nutritious principles and vitamins and renders it quite useless. This is an ideal food for Sadhakas. Milk is a perfect food by itself.

A fruit diet exercises a benign influence on the constitution. This is a natural form of diet. Fruits are very great energy-producers. Fruits and milk diet help concentration and easy mental focusing. Barley, wheat, milk and ghee promote longevity and increase power and strength. Fruit-juice and the water wherein sugar-candy is dissolved, are very good beverages. Butter mixed with sugar-candy, and almonds soaked in water can be taken. These will cool the system.

Forbidden Articles

Sour, hot, pungent and bitter preparations, salt, mustard, asafoetida, chillies, tamarind, sour curd, chutnee, meat, eggs, fish, garlic, onions, alcoholic liquors, acidic things, stale food, overripe or unripe fruits, and other articles that disagree with your system should be avoided entirely.

Rajasic food distracts the mind. It excites passion. Give up salt. It excites passion and emotion. Giving up of salt helps in controlling the tongue and thereby the mind and in developing will power also. Snakebite and scorpion-stings will have no influence on a man who has given up salt. Onions and garlic are worse than meat.

Live a natural life. Take simple food that is agreeable. You should have your own menu to suit your constitution. You are yourself the best judge to select a Sattvic diet.

The proficient in Yoga should abandon articles of food detrimental to the practice of Yoga. During intense Sadhana, milk (and ghee also) is ordained.

I have given above several articles of Sattvic nature. That does not mean that you should take all. You will have to select a few things that are easily available and suitable to you. Milk is the best food for Yogins. But even a small quantity of milk is harmful for some and may not agree with all constitutions. If one form of diet is not suitable or if you feel constipated, change the diet and try some other Sattvic articles. This is Yukti.

In the matter of food and drinks you should be a master. You should not have the least craving or sense-hankering for any particular food. You must not become a slave to any particular object.

Mitahara

Heavy food leads to Tamasic state and induces sleep only. There is a general misapprehension that a large quantity of food is necessary for health and strength. Much depends upon the power of assimilation and absorption. Generally, in the vast majority of cases, most of the food passes away undigested along with feces. Take half stomachful of wholesome food. Fill a quarter with pure water. Leave the rest free. This is Mitahara. Mitahara plays a vital part in keeping up perfect health. Almost all diseases are due to irregularity of meals, overeating and unwholesome food. Eating all things at all times like a monkey is highly dangerous. Such a man can become a Rogi (sick man) easily; but he can never become a Yogi. Hear the emphatic declaration of Lord Krishna: "Success in Yoga is not for him who eats too much or too little; nor for him who sleeps too much or too little (Gita VI-16). Again in the Sloka 18 of the same chapter, He says: "To him who is temperate in eating and in sleep and wakefulness, Yoga becomes a destroyer of misery."

A glutton cannot at the very outset have diet regulations and observe Mitahara. He must gradually practice this. First let him take less quantity twice as usual. Then instead of the usual heavy night meals, let him take fruits and milk alone for some days. In due course of time he can completely avoid the night meals and try to take fruits and milk in the daytime. Those who do intense Sadhana must take milk alone. It is a perfect food by itself. If necessary they can take some easily digestible fruits. A glutton, if he all on a sudden takes to fruit or milk diet, will desire at every moment to eat something or other. That is bad. Once again, I reiterate gradual practice is necessary.

Do not fast much. It will produce weakness in you. Occasional fasting once a month or when passion troubles you much, will suffice. During fasting you should not even think of the various articles of food. Constant thinking of the food when you fast cannot bring you the desired result. During fasting, avoid company. Live alone. Utilize your time in Yogic Sadhana. After a fast do not take any heavy food. Milk or some fruit-juice is beneficial.

Do not make much fuss about your diet. You need not advertise to everyone if you are able to pull on with a particular form of diet. The observance of such Niyamas is for your advancement in the spiritual path and giving publicity to your Sadhana will not spiritually benefit you. There are many nowadays who make it a profession to earn money and their livelihood by performing some Asana, Pranayama or by having some diet regulation such as eating only raw articles or leaves or roots. They cannot have any spiritual growth. The goal of life is Self-realization. Sadhakas should keep the goal always in view and do intense Sadhana with the prescribed methods.

The Place For Yoga Sadhana

Sadhana should be done in a secluded place. There should be no interruption by anyone. When you live in a house, a well-ventilated room should be reserved for Sadhana purposes. Do not allow anybody to enter the room. Keep it under lock and key. Do not allow even your wife, children or intimate friends to enter the room. It should be kept pure and holy. It should be free from mosquitoes, flies and lice and absolutely free from dampness. Do not keep too many things in the room. They will distract you every now and then. No surrounding noise also should disturb you. The room should not be too big, as the eyes will begin to wander.

Places of cool or temperate climate are required for Yoga Abhyasa, as you will get easily exhausted in hot place. You must select such a place where you can comfortably stay all through the year in winter, summer and rainy season. You must stick to one place throughout Sadhana period. Select a beautiful and pleasant spot where there is no disturbance, on the banks of a river, lake or sea or top of a hill where there is a nice spring and grove of trees and where milk and articles of food are easily procurable. You should select such a place where there are some other Yogic practitioners. When you see others who are devoted to Yogic practices you will diligently apply yourself to your practices. You can consult them in times of difficulties. Do not wander here and there in search of a place where you will get all conveniences. Do not change your place very often when you find some inconvenience. You must put up with it. Every place has some advantage and disadvantage. Find out a place where you have many advantages and a few disadvantages.

The following places are best suited. They are admirably adapted. Scenery is charming and spiritual vibrations are marvelous and elevating. There are several Kutirs (huts) to live in for real Abhyasis, or you can construct your own hut. Milk and other rations are available in all the places from the neighboring villages. Any solitary village on the banks of Ganga, Narmada, Yamuna, Godavari,

Krishna and Kaveri is suitable. I will tell you some important places for meditation.

Kulu Valley, Champa Valley and Srinagar in Kashmir; Banrughi Guha near Tehri; Brahmavarta near Kanpur; Joshi (Prayag) in Allahabad; Canary Caves near Bombay; Mussoorie; Mt. Abu; Nainital; Brindavan; Banares; Puri; Uttara Brindavan (14 miles from Almora); Hardwar, Rishikesh (N.Rly.); Lakshmanjhula (*3), Brahmapuri Forest (*4), Ram Guha in Brahmapuri Forest, Garuda Chatty (*4), Neelkant (*8), Vasishtha Guha (*14), Uttarkashi; Deva Prayag; Badrinarayan; Gangotri, Nasik and Nandi Hills in Mysore. (* *Distance in miles from Rishikesh*)

If you build a Kutir in a crowded place, people out of curiosity will disturb you. You will have no spiritual vibrations there. There will be a lot of other disturbances also. Again you will be without any protection if you construct your Kutir in a thick forest. Thieves and wild animals will trouble you. The question of food will arise. You must consider all these points well before you select a place for your Sadhana. If you cannot go in for such places, convert a solitary room into a forest.

Your Asana (seat) for the Yogic practices should not be too high or too low. Spread a seat of *Kusha* grass, tiger-skin or deerskin and then sit. Burn incense daily in the room. In the initial period of your Sadhana you must be very particular about all these. When you have sufficiently advanced in your practice, then you need not lay much stress on such rules.

The Time

It is stated in Gheranda Samhita that Yogic practices should not be commenced in winter, summer and rainy seasons, but only in spring and autumn. This depends upon the temperature of the particular place and the strength of the individual. Generally cool hours are best suited. In hot places you should not practice during the day. Early morning hours are suitable for Yogic practices. You should completely avoid Yoga Abhyasa in summer in those places where the temperature is hot even in winter. If you live in cool places like Kodaikanal, Ooty, Kashmir, Badrinarayan, Gangotri, etc., you can practice even during the day.

As instructed in the previous lessons you should not practice when the stomach is loaded. Generally Yogic practices should be done only after a bath. A bath is not beneficial immediately after the practices. You should not sit for Yogic practices when your mind is restless or when you are worried much.

The Age

Young boys under 18 years of age whose bodies are very tender should not have too much practice. They have a very tender body which cannot stand the exertion of Yogic exercises. Further, a youth's mind will be wandering and unsettled and so, in youth one cannot concentrate well, whereas, Yogic exercises require intense and deep concentration. In old age when all vitality is sapped by unnecessary worry, anxieties, troubles and other worldly Vyavaharas, one cannot do any spiritual practice. Yoga requires full vitality, energy, power and strength. Therefore the best period for Yoga Abhyasa is from 20 to 40 years of age. Those who are strong and healthy can take to Yogic practices even after 50.

Necessity For A Yogic Guru

In olden days the aspirants were required to live with the Guru for a number of years, so that the Guru could study the students thoroughly. The food during practice, what to practice and how, whether the students are qualified for the path of Yoga, and the temperament of the aspirants and other important items have to be considered and judged by the Guru. It is the Guru that should decide whether the aspirants are of Uttamai, Madhyama or Adhama type and fix different kinds of exercises. Sadhana differs according to the nature, capacity and qualifications of the aspirants. After understanding the theory of Yoga, you will have to learn the practice from an experienced Yogic Guru. So long as there is the world, there are books on Yoga and teachers also. You will have to search for them with Sraddha, faith, devotion and earnestness. You can get easy lessons from the Guru and practice them at home also in the initial stages of practice.

When you advance a bit, for advanced and difficult exercises you will have to stay with the Guru. The personal contact with the Guru has manifold advantages. You will be highly benefited by the spiritual magnetic aura of your Guru. For the practice of Bhakti Yoga and Vedanta you do not require a Guru by your side. After learning the Srutis for sometime from a Guru, you will have to reflect and meditate alone, in entire seclusion, whereas in Kundalini Yoga you will have to break up the Granthis and take the Kundalini from Chakra to Chakra. These are all difficult processes. The method of uniting the Apana and Prana and sending it along the Sushumna and breaking the Granthis need the help of a Guru. You will have to sit at the Guru's feet for a pretty long time. You will have to understand thoroughly the location of the Nadis, Chakras and the detailed technique of the several Yogic Kriyas.

Lay bare to your Guru the secrets of your heart and the more you do so, the greater the sympathy and help you get from your Guru. This sympathy means accession of strength to you in the straggle against sin and temptation.

"Learn thou this by discipleship, by investigation and by service. The wise, the seers of the Essence of things will instruct thee in wisdom". (Gita-IV-34)

Some do meditation for some years independently. Later on they feel actually the necessity for a Guru. They come across some obstacles in the way. They do not know how to proceed further and to obviate these impediments or stumbling blocks. Then they begin to search for a master. A stranger in a big city finds it difficult to go back to his residence in a small avenue though he has walked in the way half a dozen times. When difficulty arises even in the case of finding out the way through streets and roads how much more difficult it should be in the path of spirituality when one walks alone with closed eyes!

The aspirant gets obstacles or impediments, dangers, snares and pitfalls on the spiritual path. He may commit errors in Sadhana also. A Guru, who has already trodden the path and reached the goal, is very necessary to guide him.

Who Is A Guru?

Guru is one who has full Self-illumination and who removes the veil of ignorance in deluded Jivas. Guru, Truth, Brahman, Ishvara, Atman, God, Om are all one. The number of realized souls may be less in this Kali Yuga when compared with the Satya Yuga, but they are always present to help the aspirants. They are always searching for the proper Adhikarins.

Guru is Brahman Himself. Guru is Ishvara Himself. Guru is God. A word from him is a word from God. He need not teach any. Even his mere presence or company is elevating, inspiring and soul-stirring. The very company itself is self-illumination. Living in his company is spiritual education. That which comes out of his lips is all Vedas or gospel truth. His very life is an embodiment of Vedas. Guru is your guide or spiritual preceptor, real father, mother, brother, relative and intimate friend. He is an embodiment of mercy and love. His tender smile radiates light, bliss, joy, knowledge and peace. He is a blessing to the suffering humanity. Whatever he talks is Upanishadic teaching. He knows the spiritual path. He knows the pitfalls and snares on the way. He gives warning to the aspirants. He removes obstacles on the path. He imparts spiritual strength to the students. He showers his grace on their heads. He takes their Prarabdha even on his head. He is the ocean of mercy. All agonies, miseries, tribulations, taints of worldliness, etc., vanish in his presence.

It is he who transmutes the little Jivahood into great Brahmanhood. It is he who overhauls the old, wrong, vicious Samskaras of the aspirants and awakens them to the attainment of the knowledge of Self. It is he who uplifts the Jivas from the quagmire of body and Samsara, removes the veil of Avidya, all doubts, Moha and fear, awakens Kundalini and opens the inner eye of intuition.

The Guru must not only be a Srotriya but a Brahma-Nishtha also. Mere study of books cannot make one a Guru. One who has studied Vedas and who has direct knowledge of Atman through Anubhava can only be considered a Guru. If you can find peace in the presence of a Mahatma, and if your doubts are removed by his very presence you can take him as your Guru.

A Guru can awaken the Kundalini of an aspirant through sight, touch, speech or mere Sankalpa (thought). He can transmit spirituality to the student just as one gives an orange-fruit to another. When the Guru gives Mantra to his disciples, he gives it with his own power and Sattvic Bhava.

The Guru tests the students in various ways. Some students misunderstand him and lose their faith in him. Hence, they are not benefited. Those who stand the tests boldly come out successful in the end. The periodical examinations in the Adhyatmic University of Sages are very stiff indeed. In days of yore the tests were very severe. Once Gorakhnath asked some of his students to climb up a tall tree and throw themselves head downwards on a very sharp Trident (*Trishul*). Many faithless students kept quiet. But one faithful student at once climbed up the tree with lightning speed and threw himself down. The invisible hand of Gorakhnath protected him. He had immediate Self-realization. He had no Deha-adhyasa (attachment for his body). The other faithless students had strong Moha and Ajnana.

There is a good deal of heated debates and controversy amongst many people on the matter of the necessity of a Guru. Some of them assert with vehemence and force that a preceptor is not at all necessary for Self-realization and spiritual advancement and that one can have spiritual progress and self-illumination through one's own efforts only. They quote various passages from scriptures and assign arguments and reasonings to support them. Others boldly assert with greater emphasis and force that no spiritual progress is possible for a man, however intelligent he may be, however hard he may attempt and struggle in the spiritual path, unless he gets the benign grace and direct guidance of a spiritual preceptor.

Now open your eyes and watch carefully what is going on in this world in all walks of life. Even a cook needs a teacher. He serves under a senior cook for some years. He obeys him implicitly. He pleases his teacher in all possible ways. He learns all the techniques in cooking. He gets knowledge through the grace of his senior cook, his teacher. A junior lawyer wants the help and guidance of a senior advocate. Students of mathematics and medicine need the help and guidance of a Professor. A student of Science, music and astronomy wants the guidance of a scientist and musician and an astronomer. When such is the case with ordinary, secular knowledge, then, what to speak of the inner spiritual path, wherein the student has to walk alone with closed eyes? When you are in a thick jungle, you come across several cross footpaths. You are in a dilemma. You do not know the directions and by which path you should go. You are bewildered. You want a guide here to direct you in the right path. It is universally admitted that an efficient teacher is needed in all branches of knowledge in this physical plane and that physical, mental, moral and cultural growth can only be had through the help and guidance of a capable master. This is a universal inexorable law of nature. Why do you deny them, friend, the application of this universally accepted law in the realm of spirituality?

Spiritual knowledge is a matter of Guruparampara. It is handed down from a Guru to his disciple. Study Brihadaranyaka Upanishad. You will have a comprehensive understanding. Gaudapadacharya imparted Self-knowledge to his disciple Govindapadacharya; Govindapadacharya to his disciple Sankaracharya; Sankaracharya to his disciple Suresvaracharya. Gorakhnath to Nivrittinath; Nivrittinath to Jnanadev. Totapuri imparted knowledge to Ramakrishna; Ramakrishna to Vivekananda. It was Dr. Annie Besant who molded the career of Sri Krishnamurthi. It was Ashtavakra who molded the life of Raja Janaka. It was Gorakhnath who shaped the spiritual destiny of Raja Bhartrihari. It was Lord Krishna who made Arjuna and Uddhava establish themselves in the spiritual path, when their minds were in an unsettled condition.

Some aspirants do meditation for some years independently. Later on they feel actually the necessity for a Guru. They come across some obstacles in the way. They do not know how to proceed further and how to obviate these impediments or stumbling blocks. Then they begin to search for a Guru.

The student and the teacher should live together as father and devoted son or as a husband and wife with extreme sincerity and devotion. The aspirant should have an eager, receptive attitude to imbibe the teachings of the master. Then only will the aspirant be spiritually benefited; otherwise, there is not the least hope of the spiritual life of the aspirant and complete regeneration of his old Asuric nature.

It is a great pity that the present system of education in India is not favorable to the spiritual growth of Sadhakas. The minds of the students are saturated with materialistic poison. Aspirants of the present day have not got any idea of the true relationship of Guru and a disciple. It is not like the relationship of a student and teacher or professor in schools and colleges. Spiritual relationship is entirely different. It involves dedication. It is very sacred. It is purely divine. Turn the pages of the Upanishads. In days of yore, Brahmacharins used to approach their teachers with profound humility, sincerity and Bhava.

Spiritual Power

Just as you can give an orange to a man and take it back, so also spiritual power can be transmitted by one to another and taken back also. This method of transmitting spiritual power is termed "*Shakti Sanchara*."

Birds keep their eggs under their wings. Through heat the eggs are hatched. Fish lay their eggs and look at them. They are hatched. The tortoise lays its eggs and thinks of them. They are hatched. Even so the spiritual power is transmitted by the Guru to the disciple through touch (Sparsha) like birds, sight (Darshana) like fish, and thinking or willing (Sankalpa) like the tortoise.

The transmitter, the Yogi-Guru, sometimes enters the astral body of the student and elevates his mind through his power. The Yogi (operator) makes the subject (Chela) sit in front of him and asks him to close his eyes and then transmits his spiritual power. The subject feels the spiritual power actually passing from Muladhara Chakra higher up to the neck and top of the head.

The disciple does various Hatha Yogic Kriyas, Asanas, Pranayamas, Bandhas, Mudras, etc., by himself. The student must not restrain his *Iccha-Sakti*. He must act according to the inner Prerana (inner goading or stirring). The mind is highly elevated. The moment the aspirant closes his eyes, meditation comes by itself. Through Sakti-Sanchara Kundalini is awakened by the grace of the Guru in the disciple. Sakti Sanchara comes through Parampara. It is a hidden mystic science. It is handed down from the Guru to the disciple.

The disciple should not rest satisfied with the transmission of power from the Guru. He will have to struggle hard in Sadhana for further perfection and attainments.

Sakti Sanchara is of two kinds, viz., lower and higher. The lower one is Jada Kriya only wherein one automatically does Asanas, Bandhas and Mudras without any instructions when the Guru imparts the power to the student. The student will have to take up Sravana, Manana and Nididhyasana for perfection. He cannot depend upon the Kriya alone. This Kriya is only an auxiliary. It gives a push to the Sadhaka. A fully developed Yogi only possesses the higher kind of Shakti-Sanchara.

Lord Jesus, through touch, transmitted his spiritual power to some of his disciples (Master's Touch). Samartha Ramdas touched a prostitute. She entered into Samadhi. Sri Ramakrishna Paramahamsa touched Swami Vivekananda. Swami Vivekananda had superconscious experiences. He struggled hard for seven years more even after the touch for attaining perfection. Lord Krishna touched the blind eyes of Vilvamangal (Surdas). The inner eye of Surdas was opened. He had Bhava Samadhi. Lord Gouranga, through his touch, produced Divine intoxication in many people and converted them to his side. Even atheists danced in ecstasy in the streets by his touch and sang songs of Hari. Glory, glory to such exalted Yogic Gurus.

Chapter Four

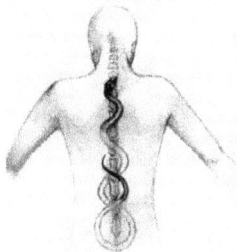

KUNDALINI YOGA — THEORY

Yoga Nadis

Nadis are the astral tubes made up of astral matter that carry psychic currents. The Sanskrit term 'Nadi' comes from the root 'Nad' which means 'motion'. It is through these Nadis (Sukshma, subtle passages), that the vital force or Pranic current moves or flows. Since they are made up of subtle matter the naked physical eyes cannot see them and you cannot make any test-tube experiments in the physical plane. These Yoga Nadis are not the ordinary nerves, arteries and veins that are known to the Vaidya Shastra (Anatomy and Physiology). Yoga Nadis are quite different from these.

The body is filled with innumerable Nadis that cannot be counted. Different authors state the number of Nadis in different ways, i.e., from 72,000 to 3,50,000. When you turn your attention to the internal structure of the body, you are struck with awe and wonder. Because the architect is the Divine Lord Himself who is assisted by skilled engineers and masons—Maya, Prakriti, Visva Karma, etc.

Nadis play a vital part in this Yoga. Kundalini when awakened will pass through Sushumna Nadi and this is possible only when the Nadis are pure. Therefore, the first step in Kundalini Yoga is the purification of Nadis. A detailed knowledge of the Nadis and Chakras is absolutely essential. Their location, functions, nature, etc., should be thoroughly studied.

The subtle lines, Yoga Nadis, have influence in the physical body. All the subtle (Sukshma) Prana, Nadis and Chakras have gross manifestation and operation in the physical body. The gross nerves and plexuses have close relationship with the subtle ones. You should understand this point well. Since the physical centers have close relationship with the astral centers, the vibrations that are produced in the physical centers by prescribed methods, have the desired effects in the astral centers.

Whenever there is an interlacing of several nerves, arteries and veins, that center is called "Plexus." The physical material plexuses that are known to the Vaidya Shastra are: — Pampiniform, Cervical, Brachial, Coccygeal, Lumbar, Sacral, Cardiac, Esophageal, Hepatic Pharyngeal, Pulmonary, Ligual Prostatic Plexus, etc. Similarly there are plexuses or centers of vital forces in the Sukshma Nadis. They are known as 'Padma' (lotus) or Chakras. Detailed instructions on all these centers are given elsewhere.

All the Nadis spring from the Kanda. It is in the junction where the Sushumna Nadi is connected with the Muladhara Chakra. Some say, that this Kanda is 12 inches above the anus. Out of the innumerable Nadis 14 are said to be important. They are: — Again Ida, Pingala and Sushumna are the most important of the above 14 Nadis, and Sushumna is the chief. It is the highest and most sought by the Yogins. Other Nadis are subordinate to this. Detailed instructions on each Nadi and its functions and the method of awakening the Kundalini and passing it from Chakra to Chakra are given in the following pages.

Spinal Column

Before proceeding to the study of Nadis and Chakras you will have to know something about the Spinal Column, as all the Chakras are connected with it. Spinal Column is known as Meru Danda. This is the axis of the body just as Mount Meru is the axis of the earth. Hence the spine is called 'Meru'. Spinal column is otherwise known as spine, axis-staff or vertebral column. Man is microcosm. (*Pinda - Kshudra-Brahmanda*). All things seen in the universe, —mountains, rivers, Bhutas, etc., exist in the body also. All the Tattvas and Lokas (worlds) are within the body.

The body may be divided into three main parts: —head, trunk and the limbs, and the center of the body is between the head and the legs. The spinal column extends from the first vertebra, Atlas bone, to the end of the trunk.

The spine is formed of a series of 33 bones called vertebrae; according to the position these occupy, it is divided into five regions: —

1. Cervical region (neck) 7 vertebrae
2. Dorsal region (back) 12 vertebrae
3. Lumbar region (waist or loins) 5 vertebrae.
4. Sacral region (buttocks, Sacrum or gluteal) 5 vertebrae.
5. Coccygeal region (imperfect vertebrae Coccyx) 4 vertebrae.

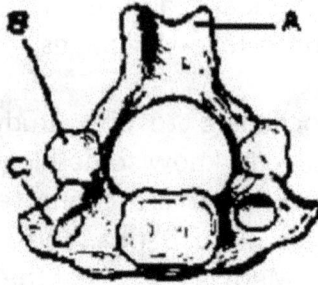

Vertebrae

The vertebral bones are piled one upon the other thus forming a pillar for the support of the cranium and trunk. They are connected together by spinous, transverse and articular processes and by pads of fibro-cartilage between the bones. The arches of the vertebrae form a hollow cylinder or a bony covering or a passage for the spinal cord. The size of the vertebrae differs from each other. For example, the size of the vertebrae in cervical region is smaller than in dorsal but the arches are bigger. The body of the lumbar vertebrae is the largest and biggest. The whole spine is not like a stiff rod, but has curvatures that give a spring action. All the other bones of the body are connected with this spine.

Between each pair of vertebrae there are apertures through which the spinal nerves pass from the spinal cord to the different portions and organs of the body. The five regions of the spine correspond with the regions of the five Chakras: Muladhara, Svadhishthana, Manipura, Anahata and Vishuddha. Sushumna Nadi passes through the hollow cylindrical cavity of the vertebral column and Ida is on the left side and Pingala on the right side of the spine.

Sukshma Sarira

The physical body is shaped in accordance with the nature of the astral body. The physical body is something like water, Sthula form. When water is heated, the steam or vapor corresponds to the astral body. In the same way the astral or Sukshma body is within the gross or physical body. The gross body cannot do anything without the astral body. Every gross center of the body has its astral center. A clear knowledge of the gross body is of utmost importance as this Yoga deals with the center of the astral body. In subsequent chapters you will find, therefore, a short description of the centers of the gross body and their corresponding centers in the Sukshma Sarira. You will find the descriptions of the astral centers and their connected functions in the physical body.

Kanda

This is situated between the anus and the root of the reproductory organ. It is like the shape of an egg and is covered with membranes. This is just above the Muladhara Chakra. All the Nadis of the body spring from this Kanda. It is in the junction where Sushumna is connected with Muladhara Chakra. The four petals of the Muladhara Chakra are on the sides of this Kanda and the junction is called Granthi-Sthana, where the influence of Maya is very strong. In some Upanishads you will find that Kanda is 9 digits above the genitals.

Kanda is a center of the astral body from where Yoga Nadis, subtle channels, spring and carry the Sukshma Prana (vital energy) to the different parts of the body. Corresponding to this center, you have 'Cauda equina' in the gross physical body. The spinal cord extending from the brain to the end of the vertebral column tapers off into a fine silken thread. Before its termination it gives off innumerable fibers, crowded into a bunch of nerves. This bunch of nerves is 'Cauda equina' in the gross body. The astral center of 'Cauda equina' is Kanda.

Spinal Cord

The central nervous system consists of the brain and the spinal cord, the cerebro-spinal center or axis. The continuation of the *Medulla oblongata* or the *Bulb* is a connecting medium between the brain and the spinal cord. The center in the *Medulla oblongata* is closely connected with the involuntary functions of breathing and swallowing. The spinal cord extends from the top of the spinal canal to the second vertebra of the coccygeal region where it tapers off into a fine silken thread, called *Filum terminale*.

The spinal cord is a column of very soft gray and white brain-matter. The white matter is arranged on the sides of the gray matter. The white matter is of medullated nerves while the gray is of nerve cells and fibers. This is not tightly fitted with the spinal canal, but suspended or dropped, as it were, into the spinal canal just like the brain in the cranial cavity. This is nourished by the membranes. Spinal cord and brain float in the cerebro-spinal fluid. The fluid prevents, therefore, any injury done to them. Further, a covering of fatty tissue protects the spinal cord. It is divided into two symmetrical halves by an anterior and posterior fissure. In the center there is a minute canal, called *canalis centralis*. Brahmanadi runs along this canal from the Muladhara to Sahasrara Chakra. It is through this Nadi, Kundalini, when awakened, passes to Brahmarandhra.

The spinal cord is not divided or separated from the brain. It is continuous with the brain. All the cranial and spinal nerves are connected with this cord. Every nerve of the body is connected with this. The organs of reproduction, micturition, digestion, blood-circulation, and respiration are all controlled by this spinal cord. Spinal cord opens out into the fourth ventricle of the brain in the *medulla oblongata*. From the fourth ventricle it runs along the third, then the fifth ventricle of the brain and finally it reaches the crown of the head, Sahasrara Chakra.

Sushumna Nadi

When we study the construction, location and function of the Spinal Cord and the Sushumna Nadi, we can readily say that the Yogins of yore called the Spinal Cord Sushumna Nadi. The Western Anatomy deals with the gross form and functions of the Spinal Cord, while the Yogins of ancient times dealt with all about the subtle (Sukshma) nature. Now in Kundalini Yoga, you should have a thorough knowledge of this Nadi.

Sushumna extends from the Muladhara Chakra (second vertebra of coccygeal region) to Brahmarandhra. The Western Anatomy admits that there is a central canal in the Spinal Cord, called *Canalis Centralis* and that the cord is made up of gray and white brain-matter. Spinal Cord is dropped or suspended in the hollow of the spinal column. In the same way, Sushumna is dropped within the spinal canal and has subtle sections. It is of red color like Agni (fire).

Within this Sushumna there is a Nadi by name Vajra which is lustrous as Surya (sun) with Rajasic qualities. Again within this Vajra Nadi, there is another Nadi, called Chitra. It is of Sattvic nature and of pale color. The qualities of Agni, Surya and Chandra (fire, sun and moon) are the three aspects of Sabda Brahman. Here within this Chitra, there is a very fine minute canal (which is known as *Canalis Centralis*). This canal is known as Brahmanadi through which Kundalini, when awakened, passes from Muladhara to Sahasrara Chakra. In   this center exist all the six Chakras (lotuses, viz.,   Muladhara, Svadhishthana, Manipura, Anahata, Vishuddha and Ajna).

The lower extremity of the Chitra Nadi is called Brahmadvara, the door of Brahman, as Kundalini has to pass through this door to Brahmarandhra. This corresponds to Haridwar which is the gate of Hari of Badrinarayan in the macrocosm (physical plane). The Chitra terminates in the Cerebellum.

In a general sense the Sushumna Nadi itself (gross Spinal Cord) is called Brahma Nadi because, Brahma Nadi is within the Sushumna. Again the canal within the Chitra is also called Sushumna, because the canal is within the Sushumna. Ida and Pingala Nadis are on the left and right sides of the spine.

Chitra is the highest and most beloved of the Yogins. It is like a thin thread of lotus. Brilliant with five colors, it is in the center of Sushumna. It is the most vital part of the body. This is called the Heavenly way. It is the giver of Immortality. By contemplating on the Chakras that exist in this Nadi, the Yogi destroys all sins and attains the Highest Bliss. It is the giver of Moksha.

When the breath flows through Sushumna, the mind becomes steady. This steadiness of the mind is termed "Unmani Avastha", the highest state of Yoga. If you sit for meditation when Sushumna is operating, you will have wonderful meditation. When the Nadis are full of impurities, the breath cannot pass into the middle Nadi. So one should practice Pranayama for the purification of Nadis.

Para-Sympathetic And Sympathetic System

On either side of the spinal cord run the sympathetic and para-sympathetic cords, a double chain of ganglia.

Ganglia means a collection of nerve cells. These constitute the Autonomic System which supplies nerves to the involuntary organs, such as heart, lungs, intestines, kidneys, liver, etc., and controls them. *Vagus* nerve, which plays a vital part in human economy, comes out of this sympathetic system. Sympathetic system stimulates or accelerates. Para-sympathetic system retards or inhibits. There are nerves to dilate or expand the arteries which carry pure oxygenated blood to nourish the tissues, organs and cells of different parts of the body. These are called *Vaso-dilators.* Filaments connect the left and the right sympathetic chains. These cross from the right to the left side and *vice versa*, but the exact places where these crosses are not known, though several have attempted to find. M'Kendrick and Snodgrass in their *Physiology of the Senses* write: "Where the sensory fibers cross from one side to the other is not known. In some parts of the spinal cord the sensory fibers do cross from the right to left side and *vice versa.*"

Ida And Pingala Nadis

Ida and Pingala Nadis are not the gross sympathetic chains. These are the subtle Nadis that carry the Sukshma Prana. In the physical body these tentatively correspond to the right and left sympathetic chains.

Ida starts from the right testicle and Pingala from the left testicle. They meet with Sushumna Nadi at the Muladhara Chakra and make a knot there. This junction of three Nadis at the Muladhara Chakra is known as Mukta Triveni. Ganga, Yamuna and Sarasvati dwell in Pingala, Ida and Sushumna Nadis respectively. This meeting place is called Brahma Granthi. Again these meet at the Anahata and Ajna Chakra. In the macrocosm also you have a Triveni at Prayag where the three rivers Ganga, Yamuna and Sarasvati meet.

Ida flows through the left nostril and Pingala through the right nostril. Ida is also called Chandra Nadi (moon) and Pingala as Surya Nadi (sun). Ida is cooling and Pingala is heating. Pingala digests the food. Ida is of pale, Sakti Rupa. It is the great nourisher of the world. Pingala is of fiery red, Rudra Rupa. Ida and Pingala indicate Kala (time) and Sushumna swallows time. The Yogi knows the time of his death; takes his Prana into Sushumna; keeps it in Brahmarandhra, and defies time (Kala—death). The famous Yogi Sri Chang Dev of Maharashtra fought against death several times by taking the Prana into Sushumna. He was a contemporary of Sri Jnanadev of Alandi, near Poona. It was he who had Bhuta Siddhi, control over wild animals, through his Yogic practices. He came on the back of a tiger to see Sri Jnanadev.

Svara Sadhana

Svara Sadhana, practice of breath, is the revealer of Satya, Brahman and bestower of the Supreme Knowledge and Bliss. Perform calm acts during the flow of Ida and harsh acts during the flow of Pingala. Do acts resulting in the attainment of psychic powers, Yoga, meditation, etc., during the flow of the Sushumna. If the breath rises by Ida (moon) at sunrise and flows throughout the day, and Pingala (sun) rises at sunset and flows throughout the night it confers considerable good results. *Let the breath flow through Ida the whole day and through Pingala the whole night. He who practices thus is verily a great Yogi.*

How To Change The Flow In Nadis

The following exercises are for changing the flow from Ida to Pingala. Select any one of the methods that suits you best. For changing the flow from Pingala to Ida, just do the same exercise on the opposite side:

1. Plug the left nostril with a small piece of cotton or fine cloth for a few minutes.

2. Lie down on the left side for ten minutes.

3. Sit erect. Draw the left knee up and keep the left heel near the left buttock. Now press the left armpit, *Axilla*, on the knee. In a few seconds the flow will be through Pingala.

4. Keep the two heels together near the right buttock. The right knee will be over the left knee. Keep the left palm on the ground a foot away and let the weight of the trunk rest on the left hand. Do not bend at the elbow. Turn the head also towards the left side. This is an effective method. Catch hold of the left ankle with the right hand.

5. The flow of breath can be changed by Nauli Kriya also.

6. There are some who are able to change the flow by will.

7. Place the *Yoga Danda* or *Hamsa Danda* (a wooden stick of about 2 feet in length with a rest of the shape of U at one end) at the left armpit and lean on it by the left side.

8. The most effective and instantaneous result is produced in changing the flow through Khechari Mudra. The Yogi turns the tongue inside and blocks the air passage by the tip of the tongue.

The above exercise is intended for general regulation of breath. Many other special exercises for the purification of Nadis and awakening Kundalini will be given in the subsequent chapters. A knowledge more secret than the science of breath, a friend more true than the science of breath, has never been seen or heard of. Friends are brought together by the power of breath. Wealth is obtained with comfort and reputation through the power of breath. The knowledge of the past, present and the future and all other Siddhis are acquired and a man reaches the highest state, by the power of breath.

I want you to practice every day the Svara Sadhana systematically and regularly, that is, to allow the flow of breath through the left nostril throughout the day and through the right nostril throughout the night. This will, doubtless, bestow on you wonderful benefits. Wrong Svara is the cause of a host of ailments. Observance of right Svara as described above leads to health and long life. Verily, verily, I say this unto you, my dear children! Practice this. Practice this from today. Shake off your habitual sloth, indolence and inertia. Leave off your idle talk. Do something practical. Before you begin the practice, pray to Lord Siva, who is the giver of this wonderful science by uttering Om Namah Sivaya and Sri Ganesha, the remover of all obstacles.

Other Nadis

Gandhari, Hastajihva, Kuhu, Sarasvati, Pusha, Sankhini, Payasvini, Varuni, Alambusha, Vishvodhara, Yasasvini, etc., are some other important Nadis. These have their origin in Kanda. All these Nadis are placed on the sides of Sushumna, Ida and Pingala, and proceed to different parts of the body to perform certain special functions. These are all subtle Nadis. Innumerable minor Nadis spring from these. As the leaf of the *Asvattha* tree is covered with minute fibers so also, this body is permeated with thousands of Nadis.

Padmas Or Chakras

Chakras are in the Linga Sarira (astral body). Linga Sarira is of 17 Tattvas, viz., 5 *Jnanendriyas* (ears, skin, eyes, tongue and nose); 5 *Karmendriyas* (speech, hands, legs, genitals, anus); 5 *Pranas* (Prana, Apana, Vyana, Udana, Samana); Manas (mind); and *Buddhi* (intellect). These have corresponding centers in the spinal cord and the nerve-plexuses in the gross body. Each Chakra has control and function over a particular center in gross body. These cannot be seen by the naked eyes. Some foolish doctors search for the Chakras in the physical body. They cannot find them there. Since they cannot find any Chakra in a dead body, they lose faith in Shastras and Yogic Kriyas.

Sukshma Prana moves in the nervous system of the Linga Sarira (astral body). Sthula Prana moves in the nervous system of the gross physical body. The two courses are intimately connected. They act and react upon each other. The Chakras are in the astral body even after the disintegration of the physical organism to death. According to a school of thought, the Chakras are formed during concentration and meditation only. This is not possible. The Chakras should exist there in a subtle state, as the gross matter is the result of the subtle matter. Without the subtle body, the gross body is impossible. The meaning of this sentence should be taken to be that one can feel and understand the Sukshma Chakras during concentration and meditation only.

Wherever there is an interlacing of several nerves, arteries and veins, that center is called Plexuses. The physical gross plexuses that are known to the Vaidya Shastra are Hepatic, Cervical, Brachial, Coccygeal, Lumbar, Sacral, Cardiac, Epigastric, Esophageal, Pharyngeal, Plumonary, Lingual, Prostatic, etc. Similarly there are plexuses or centers of Sukshma Prana in the Sushumna Nadi. All the functions of the body, nervous, digestive, circulatory, respiratory, genito-urinary and all other systems of the body are under the control of these centers in Sushumna. These are subtle centers of vital energy. These are the centers of consciousness (*Chaitanya*). These subtle centers of Sushumna have their corresponding centers in the physical body. For example, Anahata Chakra, which is in the Sushumna Nadi, has its corresponding center in the physical body at the heart (Cardiac Plexus).

The subtle centers in the Sushumna Nadi are otherwise known as Lotuses or Chakras. A particular Tattva preponderates at every Chakra. There is a presiding deity in each Chakra. In every Chakra a certain animal is represented. It denotes that the center has the qualities, Tattvas or Gunas of that particular animal. There are six important Chakras: Muladhara, Svadhisthana, Manipura, Anahata, Vishuddha, and Ajna. Sahasrara is the chief Chakra. It is in the head. These 7 Chakras correspond to the Lokas (*Bhuh, Bhuvah, Svah, Maha, Jana, Tapa, and Satya Lokas*). Muladhara to Vishuddha are the centers of *Pancha Bhutas* (five elements): earth, water, fire, air and ether.

When Kundalini is awakened it passes on from Muladhara to Sahasrara through all the Chakras. At every center to which the Yogi directs the Kundalini, he experiences a special form of Ananda (Bliss) and gains special Siddhis (psychic powers) and knowledge. He enjoys the Supreme Bliss when Kundalini is taken to Sahasrara Chakra.

The following are some other Chakras: Adhara (another name of Muladhara Chakra), Amrita, Ananda, Lalita, Balvana, Brahmadvara, Chandra, Dipaka, Karnamula, Gulhaha, Kuladipa, Kundali, Galabaddha, Kaladaada, Kaladhvara, Karangaka, Kalabhedan, Lalana, Mahotsaha, Manas, Talana, Mahapadma, Niradhara, Naukula, Prana, Soma, Triveni, Urdhvarandhra, Vajra, etc. Some of these names refer to the six important Chakras only. There are also many minor Chakras. Some Hatha yogis say, that there are 21 minor Chakras besides 13 major Chakras and some other Hatha yogis hold that there are forty-nine Chakras while the ancient Yogis taught that there are 144 Chakras. Talana Chakra with its twelve red petals is located near the base of the palate and Manas Chakra with its six petals closely associated with sensations, dreams and astral traveling. Detailed instructions of each Chakra are given in the foregoing chapters.

Petals On Chakras

Each Chakra has a particular number of petals with a Sanskrit alphabet on each petal. The corresponding Sanskrit letter represents the vibration that is produced at each petal. Every letter denotes the Mantra of Devi Kundalini. The letters exist in the petals in a latent form. These can be manifested and the vibrations of the Nadis felt during concentration.

The number of petals of the lotuses varies. Muladhara, Svadhishthana, Manipura, Anahata, Vishuddha and Ajna Chakras have 4, 6, 10, 12, 16, and 2 petals respectively. All the 50 Sanskrit letters are on the 50 petals. The number of petals in each Chakra is determined by the number and position of the Yoga Nadis around the Chakra. I will make it still clear. From each Chakra a particular number of Yoga Nadis crop up. The Chakra gives the appearance of a lotus with the Nadis as its petals. The sound produced by the vibrations of the Yoga Nadis is represented by the corresponding Sanskrit letter. The Chakras with their petals hang downwards when Kundalini is at the Muladhara Chakra. When it is awakened, they turn towards Brahmarandhra. They always face the side of Kundalini.

Muladhara Chakra

Muladhara Chakra is located at the base of the spinal column. It lies between the origin of the reproductory organ and the anus. It is just below the Kanda and the junction where Ida, Pingala and Sushumna Nadis meet. Two fingers above the anus and about two fingers below the genitals, four fingers in width is the space where the Muladhara Chakra is situated. This is the Adhara Chakra (support) as the other Chakras are above this. Kundalini, which gives power and energy to all the Chakras, lies at this Chakra. Hence this, which is the support of all, is called Muladhara or Adhara Chakra.

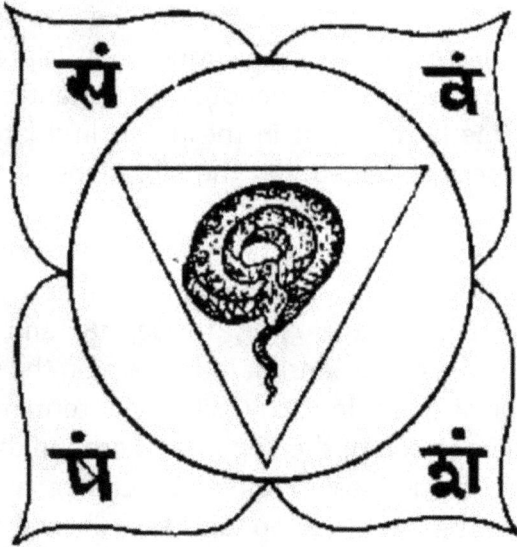

THE MULADHARA AND KUNDALINI

From this Chakra four important Nadis emanate which appear as petals of a lotus. The subtle vibrations that are made by each Nadi are represented by the Sanskrit letters: v:ö S:ö \:ö and s:ö (vaü, ÷aü, ùaü,and saü.). The Yoni that is in the center of this Chakra is called Kama and it is worshipped by Siddhas. Here Kundalini lies dormant. Ganesa is the Devata of this Chakra. The seven underworlds: *Atala, Vitala, Sutala, Talatala, Rasatala, Mahatala* and *Patala Lokas* are below this Chakra. This Chakra corresponds with *Bhu* Loka or *Bhu-Mandal,* physical plane (region of earth). *Bhuvah, Svah* or *Svarga, Maha, Jana,*

Tapa and *Satya* Lokas are above this Chakra. All the underworlds refer to some minor Chakras in the limbs which are controlled by the Muladhara Chakra. That Yogi, who has penetrated this Chakra through Prithvi Dharan, has conquered the Prithvi Tattva. He has no fear of death from earth. Prithvi is of yellow color. The golden Tripura (fire, sun and moon) is termed the 'Bija'. It is also called the great energy (Param *Tejas*) which rests on the Muladhara Chakra and which is known as Svayambhu Linga. Near this Linga is the golden region known as Kula and the presiding deity is Dakini (Shakti). Brahma Granthi or the knot of Brahma is in this Chakra. Vishnu Granthi and Rudra Granthi are in the Anahata and Ajna Chakras. l:ö (*laü*) is the Bija of Muladhara Chakra.

The wise Yogi, who concentrates and meditates on the Muladhara Chakra, acquires the full knowledge of Kundalini and the means to awaken it. When Kundalini is awakened, he gets Darduri Siddhi, the power to rise from the ground. He can control the breath, mind and semen. His Prana enters the middle Brahma Nadi. All his sins are destroyed. He acquires knowledge of the past, present and future. He enjoys the natural Bliss (Sahaja Ananda).

Svadhishthana Chakra

Svadhishthana Chakra is located within the Sushumna Nadi at the root of the reproductory organ. This corresponds to Bhuvar Loka. This has control over the lower abdomen, kidneys, etc., in the physical body. *Jala Mandal* (region of water—Apa Tattva) is here. Within this Chakra there is a space like a crescent moon or the form of a conch or *Kunda* flower. The presiding deity is Lord Brahma and Devata is Goddess Rakini. Bijakshara v:ö (vaü), the Bija of Varuna, is in this Chakra. The color of the Chakra is pure blood-like red or the color of *Sindura* (vermilion). From this center six Yoga Nadis emanate, which appear like the petals of a lotus. The vibrations that are produced by the Nadis are represented by the Sanskrit letters: *baü bhaü maü yaü raü* and *laü*.

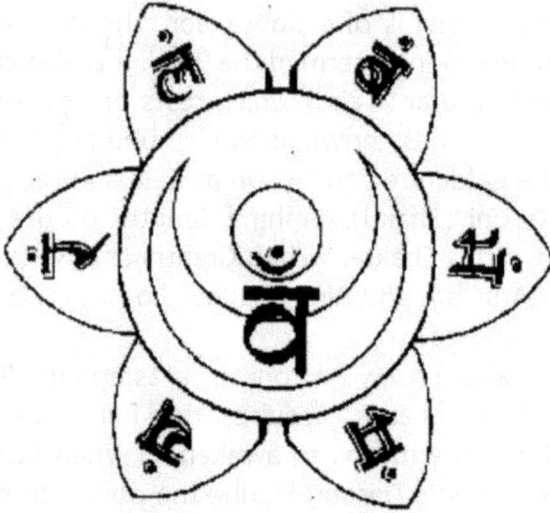

SVADHISHTHANA CHAKRA

He who concentrates at this Chakra and meditates on the Devata has no fear of water. He has perfect control over the water element. He gets many psychic powers, intuitional knowledge and a perfect control over his senses. He has full knowledge of the astral entities. Kama, Krodha, Lobha, Moha, Mada, Matsarya and other impure qualities are completely annihilated. The Yogi becomes the conqueror of death (*Mrityunjaya*).

Manipura Chakra

Manipura is the third Chakra from the Muladhara. It is located within the Sushumna Nadi, in the Nabhi Sthana (region of navel). This has its corresponding center in the physical body and has control over the liver, stomach, etc. This is a very important center. From this Chakra emanate ten Yoga Nadis which appear like the petals of a lotus. The vibrations that are produced by the Nadis are represented by the Sanskrit letters: óaü óhaü õaü taü thaü daü dhaü naü paü and phaü. The Chakra is of the color of dark clouds. Within there is a space triangular in form. It is the Agni Mandala (region of fire—Agni Tattva). The Bijakshara raü, the Bija of Agni, is here. The presiding deity is Vishnu and Goddess is Lakshmi. This Chakra corresponds to Svah or Svarga Loka and to Solar Plexus in the physical body.

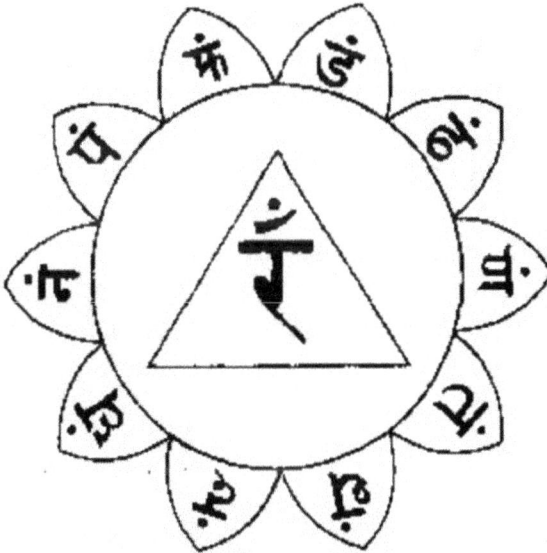

MANIPURA CHAKRA

The Yogi who concentrates at this Chakra gets Patala Siddhi, can acquire hidden treasures and will be free from all diseases. He has no fear at all from Agni (fire). "Even if he is thrown into the burning fire, he remains alive without fear of death." (*Gheranda Samhita*).

Anahata Chakra

Anahata Chakra is situated in the Sushumna Nadi (Sukshma center). It has control over the heart. It corresponds to the Cardiac Plexus in the physical body. This corresponds to Mahar Loka. The Chakra is of deep red color. Within this Chakra there is a hexagonal space of smoke or deep black color or the color of collyrium (used for the eyes). This chakra is the center of Vayu Mandal (region of air, Vayu Tattva). From here 15 Yoga Nadis emanate. The sound that is produced by each Nadi is represented by the following Sanskrit letters: kaü khaü gaü ghaü ïaü caü chaü jaü jhaü ¤aü ñaü and ñhaü. The Bijakshara yaü, the Bija of Vayu, is here. The presiding deity is Isha (Rudra) and Devata is Kakini. In the Muladhara Chakra there is Svayambhu Linga and in Anahata Chakra we have Bana Linga. Kalpa Vriksha, which gives all the desired things, is here. Anahata sound, the sound of Shabda Brahman, is heard at this center. When you do Sirshasana for a long time, you can distinctly hear this sound. Vayu Tattva is full of Sattva Guna. Vishnu Granthi is in this Sthana.

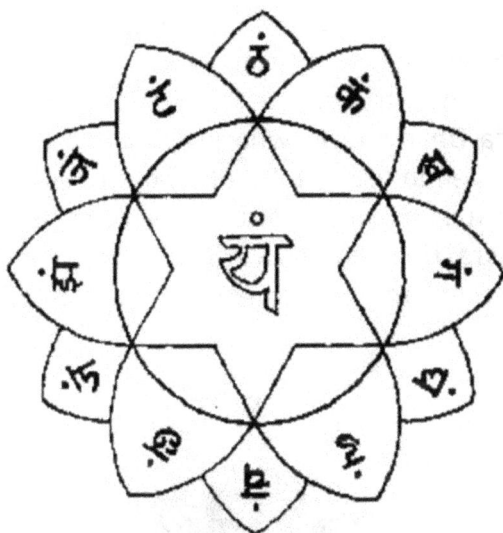

ANAHATA CHAKRA

He who meditates on this Chakra has full control over Vayu Tattva. He gets *Bhuchari Siddhi, Khechari Siddhi, Kaya Siddhi,* etc., (flying in air, entering the body of another). He gets cosmic love and all other divine Sattvic qualities.

Vishuddha Chakra

Vishuddha Chakra is situated within the Sushumna Nadi at the base of the throat, *Kantha-Mula Sthana.* This corresponds to Janar Loka. It is the center of Akasa Tattva (ether element). The Tattva is of pure blue color. Above this, all other Chakras belong to Manas Tattva. The presiding deity is Sadasiva (Isvara Linga), and the Goddess is Shakini. From this center emanate 16 Yoga Nadis which appear like the petals of a lotus. The vibrations that are produced by the Nadis are represented by the 16 Sanskrit vowels: aü àü iü ãü uü åü çü éü ëü íü eü aiü oü auü aü and aþ. Akasa Mandal (the region of ether) is round in shape like the full moon. The Bija of Akasa Tattva haü is in this center. It is of white color. This Chakra corresponds to Laryngeal plexus in the physical body.

The concentration on the Tattva of this Chakra is called Akasa Dharana. He who practices this Dharana will not perish even in Pralaya. He attains the highest success. He gets the full knowledge of the four Vedas by meditating on this Chakra. He becomes a *Trikala Jnani* (who knows the past, the present and the future).

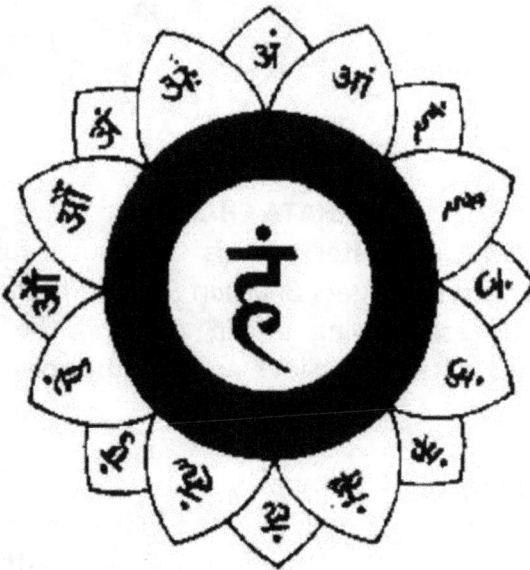

VISHUDDHA CHAKRA

Ajna Chakra

Ajna Chakra is situated within the Sushumna Nadi and its corresponding center in the physical body is at the space between the two eyebrows. This is known as Trikuti. The presiding deity, Paramasiva (Shambhu), is in the form of Hamsa. There is Goddess Hakini (Sakti). Pranava (Om) is the Bijakshara for this Chakra. This is the seat of the mind. There are two petals (Yoga Nadis) on each side of the lotus

(Chakra) and the vibrations of these Nadis are represented by the Sanskrit letters: *Ham* and *Ksham*. This is the Granthi Sthana (Rudra Granthi). The Chakra is of pure white color or like that of the full moon (on the Purnima day). Bindu, Nada and Sakti are in this Chakra. This Chakra corresponds to Tapo-Loka. The corresponding center in the physical body is at the Cavernous Plexus.

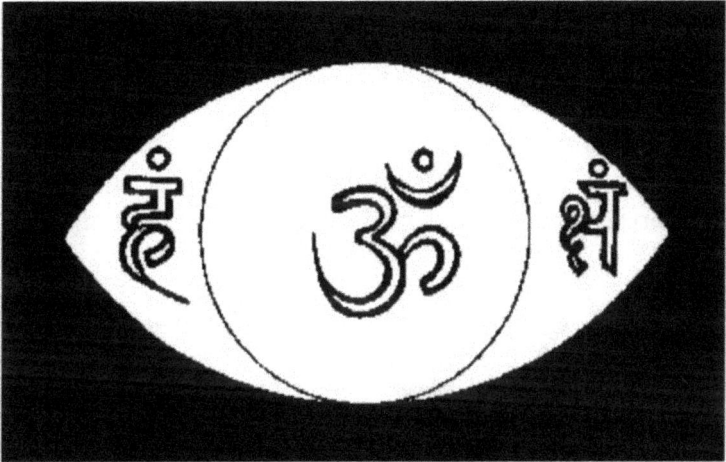

AJNA CHAKRA

He who concentrates at this center destroys all the Karmas of the past lives. The benefits that are derived by meditation on this Chakra cannot be described in words. The practitioner becomes a Jivanmukta (liberated man while living). He acquires all the 8 major and 32 minor Siddhis. All Yogis and Jnanis too concentrate to this center on the Bijakshara, Pranava! (OM). This is called Bhrumadya Drishti (gaze at the space between the two eye-brows). More details of this important Chakra will be given in the subsequent lessons.

The Brain

Brain and cranial nerves are the chief parts of the whole nervous system. It is a mass of nervous tissues made up of soft gray and white matter. It occupies the whole of cranium. Cranium is like the iron safe to keep up the treasure 'brain'. It is surrounded by three membranes or *Meninges, viz.,* (1) *dura mater,* the fibrous connective tissue by the side of the cranial bones; (2) *pia mater,* the connective tissue containing a network of blood vessels, which penetrates and nourishes all the parts of the brain; and (3) *arachnoid,* a very fine membrane around the brain. Below the *arachnoid* there is the space which contains the cerebro-spinal fluid that is intended to prevent any injury to the brain. The brain looks as if it is floating on this liquid.

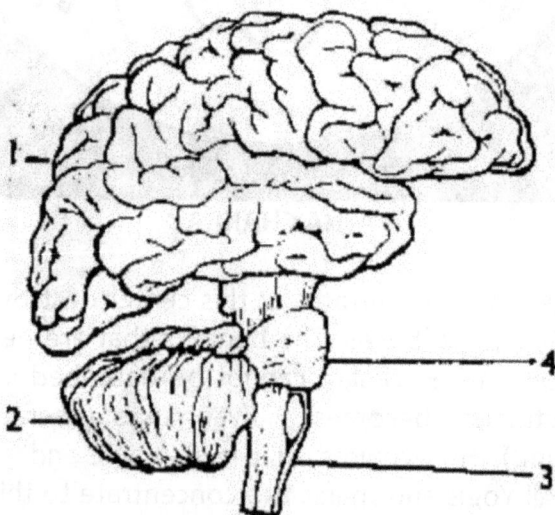

THE BRAIN

The brain can be divided into two halves, right and left hemispheres, by a central *Sulcus* or tissue. There are several lobes or smaller portions in the brain such as the parietal and temporal lobes on the sides, the occipital lobe at the posterior portion of cerebellum, etc. There are many convolutions or *Gyre* in every lobe. Again, for the sake of study, we can divide the brain into four sections.

1. *Cerebrum*: It is the anterior, oval-shaped larger part of the brain. It is situated in the upper portion of the cranial cavity. This contains the important centers of hearing, speech, sight, etc. The pineal gland which is regarded as the seat of the soul and which plays a prominent part in Samadhi and psychic phenomena is situated here.

2. *Cerebellum*, the little or hindbrain: This is the main portion of the brain, oblong-shaped, situated just above the fourth ventricle and below and behind the brain. Here the gray matter is arranged over the white matter. It regulates the muscular co-ordination. Mind rests here during dreams.

3. *Medulla Oblongata*: It is the beginning place of the spinal cord at the cranial cavity, where it is oblong-shaped and wide. It is between the two hemispheres. Here the white matter is placed over the gray matter. This contains the centers of important functions such as circulatory, respiratory, etc. This portion must be carefully protected.

4. *Pons Varolii*: It is the bridge that lies before the *Medulla Oblongata*. It is made of white and gray fibers that come from *cerebellum* and *medulla*. This is the junction where cerebellum and medulla meet.

There are five ventricles of the brain. The fourth is the most important one. It is situated in *Medulla Oblongata*. The fourth ventricle is the name of the central canal of the spinal cord, "*Canalis Centralis*" when it enters the cranial cavity. Here the tiny canal becomes bigger in size.

Every nerve of the body is closely connected with the brain. The 12 pairs of cranial nerves proceed from both hemispheres through the openings at the base of the skull to different parts of the body: Olfactory; Optic; Motor Oculi; Pathetic; Trifacial; Abducens; Facial; Auditory; Glossopharyngeal; Pneumogastric, Spinal accessory; and Hypo-glossal. These are the nerves that are connected with the eye, ear, tongue, nose, pharynx, thorax, etc. For a detailed study of this section refer to any book on anatomy. Here I have given you portions that are connected with Kundalini Yoga.

Brahmarandhra

"*Brahmarandhra*" means the hole of Brahman. It is the dwelling house of the human soul. This is also known as "*Dasamadvara*," the tenth opening or the tenth door. The hollow place in the crown of the head known as *anterior fontanelle* in the newborn child is the Brahmarandhra. This is between the two parietal and occipital bones. This portion is very soft in a babe. When the child grows, the growth of the bones of the head obliterates it. Brahma created the physical body and entered (*Pravishat*) the body to give illumination inside through this Brahmarandhra. In some of the Upanishads, it is stated like that. This is the most important part. It is very suitable for Nirguna Dhyana (abstract meditation). When the Yogi separates himself from the physical body at the time of death, this Brahmarandhra bursts open and Prana comes out through this opening (*Kapala Moksha*). "A hundred and one are the nerves of the heart. Of them one (Sushumna) has gone out piercing the head; going up through it, one attains immortality" (Kathopanishad).

Sahasrara Chakra

Sahasrara Chakra is the abode of Lord Siva. This corresponds to Satya Loka. This is situated at the crown of the head. When Kundalini is united with Lord Siva at the Sahasrara Chakra, the Yogi enjoys the Supreme Bliss, Parama Ananda. When Kundalini is taken to this center, the Yogi attains the superconscious state and the Highest Knowledge. He becomes a *Brahmavidvarishtha* or a full-blown Jnani.

The word *Sahasradala-Padma* denotes that this Padma has 1000 petals. That is, one thousand Yoga Nadis emanate from this center. There are different opinions about the exact number of petals. It is quite sufficient if you know that innumerable Nadis proceed from this center. As in the case of other Chakras, the vibrations that are made by the Yoga Nadis are represented by the Sanskrit letters. All the 50 letters of the Sanskrit alphabet are repeated here again and again on all Yoga Nadis. This is a Sukshma center. The corresponding center in the physical body is in the brain.

The term "Shat-Chakras" refers only to the chief six Chakras, *viz.*, Muladhara, Svadhishthana, Manipura, Anahata, Vishuddha and Ajna. Above all these we have Sahasrara Chakra. This is the chief of all the Chakras. All the Chakras have their intimate connection with this center. Hence this is not included as one among the Shat-Chakras. This is situated above all the Chakras.

Lalana Chakra

Lalana Chakra is situated at the space just above Ajna and below Sahasrara Chakra. Twelve Yoga Nadis emanate from this center. The vibrations that are made by the 12 Nadis are represented by the Sanskrit letters: (*Ha, Sa, Ksha, Ma, La, Va, Ra, Ya, Ha, Sa, Kha* and *Phrem*). It has OM as its Bija. At this center the Yogi concentrates on the form of his Guru and obtains all knowledge. This has control over the 12 pairs of nerves that proceed from the brain to the different sense organs.

Summary Of The Previous Lessons

Aspirants must have all the Sattvic qualities and should be quite free from impurities. Satsanga, seclusion, dietetic discipline, good manners, good character, Brahmacharya, Vairagya, etc., form the strong foundation of Yogic life. The help of a Guru, who has already trodden the path, is absolutely necessary for quick progress in the spiritual path. Places of cool, temperate climate are required for Yoga Abhyasa.

Nadis are the Sukshma (astral) channels through which Prana (vital energy) flows to different parts of the body. Ida, Pingala and Sushumna are the most important of the innumerable Nadis. All Nadis start from the Kanda. Kanda is located in the space between the origin of the reproductory organ and the anus. Sushumna Nadi is situated within the Spinal Column, in the spinal canal. Within the Sushumna Nadi there is a Nadi by name Vajra. Chitra Nadi, a minute canal, which is also called Brahmanadi, is within this Vajra Nadi. Kundalini, when awakened, passes through Chitra Nadi. These are all Sukshma centers and you cannot have any laboratory tests and test-tube experiments. Without these subtle centers, the gross physical body cannot exist and function. Muladhara, Svadhishthana, Manipura, Anahata, Vishuddha, Ajna and Sahasrara are the important Chakras. When Kundalini passes on from Chakra to Chakra, layer after layer of the mind becomes opened and the Sadhaka enters into higher states of consciousness. At every Chakra he gets various Siddhis. Ida, Pingala and other Nadis are on the sides of the spine. Ida flows through the left nostril and Pingala through the right nostril. In Svara Sadhana the breath should flow by the left nostril throughout the day and by the right nostril throughout the night.

The Mysterious Kundalini

Manastvam Vyoma tvam Marudasi Marutsarathirasi,
Tvamapastvam Bhumistvayi parinatayam nahi param,
Tvameva Svatmanam parinamayitum visvavapusha
Chidanandakaram haramahishi-bhavena bibhrushe.

"O Devi! Thou art the mind, the sky, the air, the fire, the water, and the earth. Nothing is outside Thee on Thy transformation. Thou hast become Siva's consecrated queen to alter Thy own blissful conscious Form in the shape of the world".

Kundalini, the serpent power or mystic fire, is the primordial energy or Sakti that lies dormant or sleeping in the Muladhara Chakra, the center of the body. It is called the serpentine or annular power on account of serpentine form. It is an electric fiery occult power, the great pristine force which underlies all organic and inorganic matter.

Kundalini is the cosmic power in individual bodies. It is not a material force like electricity, magnetism, centripetal or centrifugal force. It is a spiritual potential Sakti or cosmic power. In reality it has no form. The Sthula Buddhi and mind have to follow a particular form in the beginning stage. From this gross form, one can easily, understand the subtle formless Kundalini. Prana, Ahamkara, Buddhi, Indriyas, mind, five gross elements, and nerves are all the products of Kundalini.

It is the coiled-up, sleeping Divine Sakti that lies dormant in all beings. You have seen in the Muladhara Chakra that there is Svayambhu Linga. The head of the

Linga is the space where Sushumna Nadi is attached to the Kanda. This mysterious Kundalini lies face downwards at the mouth of Sushumna Nadi on the head of Svayambhu Linga. It has three and a half coils like a serpent. When it is awakened, it makes a hissing sound like that of a serpent beaten with a stick, and proceeds to the other Chakra through the Brahma Nadi, which is also called Chitra Nadi within Sushumna. Hence Kundalini is also called Bhujangini, serpent power. The three coils represent the three Gunas of Prakriti: Sattva, Rajas and Tamas, and the half represents the Vikritis, the modification of Prakriti.

Kundalini is the Goddess of speech and is praised by all. She Herself, when awakened by the Yogin, achieves for him the illumination. It is She who gives Mukti and Jnana for She is Herself that. She is also called Sarasvati, as She is the form of Sabda Brahman. She is the source of all Knowledge and Bliss. She is pure consciousness itself. She is Brahman. She is Prana Sakti, the Supreme Force, the Mother of Prana, Agni, Bindu and Nada. It is by this Sakti that the world exists. Creation, preservation and dissolution are in Her. Only by her Sakti, the world is kept up. It is through Her Sakti on subtle Prana, Nada is produced. While you utter a continuous sound or chant Dirgha Pranava! (OM), you will distinctly feel that the real vibration starts from the Muladhara Chakra. Through the vibration of this Nada, all the parts of the body function. She maintains the individual soul through the subtle Prana. In every kind of Sadhana the Goddess Kundalini is the object of worship in some form or the other.

Kundalini has connection with subtle Prana. Subtle Prana has connection with the subtle Nadis and Chakras. Subtle Nadis have connection with the mind. Mind has connection all through the body. You have heard that there is mind in every cell of the body. Prana is the working force of the body. It is dynamic. This static Sakti is affected by Pranayama and other Yogic practices and becomes dynamic. These two functions, static and dynamic, are termed 'sleeping' and 'awakening' of the Kundalini.

Chapter Five

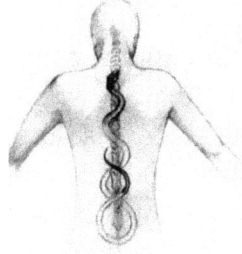

YOGA SADHANA

How To Awaken The Kundalini

One should become perfectly desireless and should be full of Vairagya before attempting to awaken Kundalini. It can be awakened only when a man rises above *Kama, Krodha, Lobha, Moha, Mada* and other impurities. Kundalini can be awakened through rising above desires of the senses. Awakening Kundalini will benefit the Yogi, who has got a pure heart and a mind free from passions and desires. If a man with a lot of impurities in the mind awakens the Sakti by sheer force through Asanas, Pranayamas and Mudras, he will break his legs and stumble down. He will not be able to ascend the Yogic ladder. This is the chief reason for people going out of the way or getting some bodily infirmities. There is nothing wrong in the Yoga. People must have purity first; then a thorough knowledge of the Sadhana, a proper guide, and a steady, gradual practice. When Kundalini is awakened there are many temptations on the way, and a Sadhaka without purity will not have the strength to resist.

A thorough knowledge of the theory is as essential as the practice. Some are of opinion that theory is not at all necessary. They bring one or two rare instances to prove that Kundalini has been awakened even in those who do not know anything about Nadis, Chakras and Kundalini. It might be due to the grace of a Guru or by mere chance. Everyone cannot expect this and neglect the theoretical side. If you look at the man in whom Kundalini has been awakened through the grace of a Guru, you will not at once begin to neglect the practical side and actually waste your time in passing from one Guru to the other. The man, who has a clear knowledge of the theory and a steady practice, attains the desired goal quickly.

Kundalini can be awakened by Pranayama, Asanas and Mudras by Hatha Yogis; by concentration and training of the mind by Raja Yogis; by devotion and perfect self-surrender by Bhaktas; by analytical will by the Jnanis; by Mantras by the Tantrikas; and by the grace of the Guru (Guru Kripa) through touch, sight or mere Sankalpa. Rousing of Kundalini and its union with Siva at the Sahasrara Chakra effect the state of Samadhi and Mukti. No Samadhi is possible without awakening the Kundalini.

For a selected few, any one of the above methods is quite sufficient to awaken the Kundalini. Many will have to combine different methods. This is according to the growth and position of the Sadhakas in the spiritual path. The Guru will find out the real position of the Sadhaka and will prescribe a proper method that will successfully awaken the Kundalini in a short period. This is something like the doctor prescribing a proper medicine to a patient to cure a particular disease. One kind of medicine will not cure the diseases of different patients. So also, one kind of Sadhana may not suit all.

There are many persons nowadays who foolishly imagine that they have attained purity, commit errors in selecting some methods and neglect many important items of Sadhana. They are poor, self-deluded souls. Self-assertive, Rajasic Sadhakas will select some exercises of their own fancy in an irregular manner and leave all the exercises when they get some serious troubles.

After Kundalini is awakened, Prana passes upwards through Brahma Nadi along with mind and Agni. You will have to take it up to Sahasrara Chakra through some special exercises such as Mahabheda, Sakti Chalana, etc.

As soon as it is awakened, it pierces the Muladhara Chakra (Bheda). It should be taken to Sahasrara through various Chakras. When Kundalini is at one Chakra, intense heat is felt there and when it leaves that center for another Chakra, the former Chakra becomes very cold and appears lifeless.

Freedom from Kama, Krodha, Raga and Dvesha and possession of balance of mind, cosmic love, astral vision, supreme fearlessness, desirelessness, Siddhis, divine intoxication and spiritual Ananda are the signs to denote the awakening of Kundalini. When it is at rest, a man has full consciousness of the world and its surroundings. When it is awakened he is dead to the world. He has no body-consciousness. He attains *Unmani* state. When Kundalini travels from Chakra to Chakra, layer after layer of the mind becomes opened and the Yogi acquires psychic powers. He gets control over the five elements. When it reaches the Sahasrara Chakra, he is in the Chidakasa (knowledge space).

Awakening of the Kundalini Sakti, its union with Siva, enjoying the nectar and other functions of the Kundalini Yoga that are described in the Yoga Sastras are misrepresented and taken in a literal sense by many. They think that they are Siva and ladies to be Sakti and that mere sexual union is the aim of Kundalini Yoga. After having some wrong interpretation of the Yogic texts, they begin to offer flowers and worship their wives with lustful propensities. The term "Divine intoxication that is derived by drinking the nectar" is also misrepresented. They take a lot of wine and other intoxicating drinks and imagine to have enjoyed the Divine ecstasy. It is mere ignorance. They are utterly wrong. This sort of worship and union is not at all Kundalini Yoga. They divert their concentration on sexual centers and ruin themselves. Some foolish young boys practice one or two Asanas, Mudras and a little Pranayama too for a few days, in any way they like, and imagine that the Kundalini has gone up to their neck. They pose as big Yogis. They are pitiable, self-deluded souls. Even a Vedanti (a student of Jnana Yoga) can get Jnana Nishtha only through awakening of the Kundalini Sakti that lies dormant at the Muladhara Chakra. No superconscious state or Samadhi is possible without awakening this primordial energy, whether it is Raja Yoga, Bhakti Yoga, Hatha Yoga or Jnana Yoga.

It is easy to awaken the Kundalini, but it is very difficult to take it to Sahasrara Chakra through the different Chakras. It demands a great deal of patience, perseverance, purity and steady practice. The Yogi, who has taken it to Sahasrara Chakra, is the real master of all forces. Generally Yogic students stop their Sadhana halfway on account of false Tushti (satisfaction). They imagine that they have reached the goal when they get some mystic experiences and psychic powers. They desire to demonstrate such powers to the public to get Khyati (reputation and fame) and to earn some money. This is a sad mistake. Full realization alone can give the final liberation, perfect peace and Highest Bliss.

Different methods of awakening the Kundalini by Hatha Yoga, Bhakti Yoga, Raja Yoga and Jnana Yoga will be described one by one. Some aspirants will not get perfection by only one method. A harmonious combination of all methods is necessary for the vast majority of persons. In the following pages I will tell you the different exercises that are intended to awaken the Kundalini. If you are wise enough, after a perusal of the different exercises, you can easily pick up the right method of Sadhana that suits you best and attain success.

Rousing of Kundalini and its union with Siva at the Sahasrara Chakra effect the state of Samadhi and Mukti. Before awakening the Kundalini, you must have Deha Suddhi (purity of body), Nadi Suddhi (purification of Nadis), Manas-Suddhi (purity of mind) and Buddhi Suddhi (purity of intellect). For the purification of the body, the following six exercises are prescribed:

Dhauti, Basti, Neti, Nauli, Tratak and Kapalabhati. These are known as Shat-Karma or the six purificatory exercises in Hatha Yoga.

1. Dhauti

Purification is of two kinds: Antar-Dhauti (internal cleaning) and Bahir-Dhauti (external cleaning). Antar-Dhauti can be made in three ways. Take a fine piece of muslin cloth, 3 inches wide and 15 feet long. The borders should be stitched well and no pieces of loose thread should be hanging from its sides. Wash it with soap before use and make it clean. Dip it in tepid water. Squeeze out the water and swallow one end of it little by little. On the first day swallow only one foot. Keep it there for a few seconds and then take it out very slowly. On the next day swallow a little more and keep it for a few minutes and then take it out slowly. Thus little by little you can swallow the whole length, retain it for about 5 minutes and then take it out. Do not be hasty. Do not injure your throat by rough handling. When the Kriya is over drink a cup of milk. This is a sort of lubrication for the throat. This exercise should be done when your stomach is empty. Morning time is good.

You need not practice this every day. Once in 4 days or a week is sufficient. This exercise cannot at all do any harm if gradually practiced. Everyone will feel a little vomiting sensation on the first 2 or 3 attempts. As soon as the Kriya is over, wash the cloth with soap and keep it always clean. This is an excellent exercise for those who are of a flabby and phlegmatic constitution. Gradual steady practice cures Gulma, gastritis, dyspepsia, diseases of the stomach and spleen, disorder of phlegm and bile. This exercise is also known as Vastra Dhauti. This is one variety of Antar-Dhauti.

There are some people who can drink plenty of water and pass it through the anus immediately. It is called Varisara Dhauti. This is an effective method. This exercise is also known as 'Sang Pachar Kriya'. Yogi Sambhunathaji of Kishkindha is an expert in this Kriya. This is not possible for the vast majority of persons. Nauli and Uddiyana Bandha should be combined for performing this exercise. Even the smoke of a cigarette can be passed out through the anus.
Drink a large quantity of water and shake the abdominal portions. Contract the stomach and vomit the water. This exercise goes with the name 'Kunjara Kriya'. This is also a kind of purificatory exercise.

Internal cleaning can be made also by swallowing air. Fill up the stomach with plenty of air. It is done by hiccough. Just as you swallow food little by little, so also you can swallow air and fill up the stomach and intestines. You will have to learn this from the man who can do this Kriya. When you contract the abdominal muscles, the air will pass away through the anus as Apana Vayu. Those who can fill up their stomach with air can float on water just like a dead body and can also live on air and water alone for some days without any food. Those who can do Antar-Dhauti in any way, need not go in for any purgative or laxative. They will never suffer from indigestion or constipation.

There are some other Dhautis, viz., Danta Dhauti (cleaning the teeth), Jihva Dhauti (cleaning the tongue), Karna Dhauti (cleaning the ears), Mula Sodhana Dhauti (cleaning the anus), etc. You all are doing these everyday. I need not tell you much about these.

2. Basti

'Basti' exercise is intended to serve the purpose of 'enema' to pass out the accumulation of feces from the intestinal canal. There are two varieties, viz., Sthala Basti and Jala Basti.

STHALA BASTI: Sit on the ground and catch hold of your toes with fingers. Do not bend the knees. This is exactly like the Paschimottanasana, but here you need not bring your head to the knees. Assuming this posture, churn the abdominal muscles and dominal muscles and expel the water. It cures uriter muscles. This is Sthala Basti.

JALA BASTI: This is more effective than Sthala Basti. Take a small bamboo tube, five inches long. Lubricate one end of it with vaseline, oil or soap. Sit in a tub of water or in a tank in knee-level of water in Utkatasana. Insert the bamboo tube about 2 or 3 inches into the anus. Contract the anus. Draw the water into the intestines slowly. Shake the abdominal muscles and expel the water. It cures urinary troubles, dropsy, constipation, etc. You should not do this everyday and make it a habit. This is only for occasional use. Do this in the morning hours before taking meals. If you do not know how to draw in the water through the tube, then you can use the ordinary syringe that is available in the market. By the use of the bamboo, you will know the method of drawing water through the anus. But in the enema syringe, water is being pushed in by the help of air. That is only the difference but the result is the same in both cases. By using the bamboo tube you can have mastery over the intestinal muscles by drawing in and pushing out the water at your command.

3. Neti

'Neti' exercise is intended for the purification of the nostrils. The nostrils must be kept always clean. Unclean nostrils will lead you to irregular breathing. Irregular breathing will make you sick.

Take a fine piece of thread about 12 inches long. There should not be any knot in the middle of the thread. It should not be too thin and weak. Insert one end of it into the right nostril and catch hold of the other end firmly. Make a forcible, continuous inhalation and pass it inside. Then slowly pull it out. Again in the same way pass it through the left nostril and take it out slowly. Do not injure your nostrils through violent pulling. After some practice, pass the thread through one nostril and take it out through the other. In the beginning you will begin to sneeze profusely when you insert the thread into the nose. This passes off after 3 or 4 attempts. This can be practiced when you find that your nostril is blocked from cold.

There is another easy method of cleaning the nostrils. Take some cold water in your hand or in a wide-mouthed cup. Draw the water slowly through the nose and expel it forcibly through the nose. There are many who can do this quite easily. After one or two attempts some persons may suffer from slight cold and cough when they begin to learn this. As soon as they are all right, again, they can practice.

You have seen many who draw the smoke of a cigarette through the mouth and pass it by the nose quite easily. If cigarette users try, they can draw the smoke through one nostril and pass it out by the other nostril or by the mouth. In the same way water also can be passed quite easily.

Drawing water and expelling it through the nose is known as 'Seet-Krama'. If you draw water through the nose and expel it through the mouth, it is called 'Vyut-Krama'. In Gheranda Samhita it is stated that this Neti Kriya purifies the skull and produces clairvoyance (Divya Drishti). Rhinitis and coryza are also cured thereby.

4. Nauli

Nauli Kriya is intended for regenerating, invigorating and stimulating the abdominal viscera and the gastro-intestinal or alimentary system. For the practice of Nauli you should know the Uddiyana Bandha. Uddiyana can be done even in a sitting posture; but Nauli is generally done while standing.

Stage I: Do a strong and forcible expiration through the mouth and keep the lungs completely empty. Contract and forcibly draw the abdominal muscles towards the back. This is Uddiyana Bandha. This is the first stage of Nauli. Uddiyana Bandha terminates in Nauli.

For practicing Nauli, stand up. Keep the right leg a foot apart from the left leg. If you keep up the feet close together, at times you may lose the balance and stumble down. Rest your hands on the thighs, thus making a slight curve of the back. Then do Uddiyana Bandha. Do this for one week before proceeding to the next stage.

Stage II: Now allow the center of the abdomen free by contracting the left and right side of the abdomen. You will have all the muscles in the center in a vertical line. This is called Madhyama Nauli. Keep it as long as you can with comfort. Do only this much for a few days.

Stage III: Here you should contract the right side of the abdomen and allow the left side free. You will have the muscles on the left side only. This is called Vama Nauli. Again contract the left side muscles and allow the right side free. This is Dakshina Nauli. By having such gradual practices, you will understand how to contract the muscles of the central, left and right sides of the abdomen. You will also notice how they move from side to side. In this stage you will see the abdominal muscles only in the central, right or the left side. Practice this stage for a week.

Stage IV: Keep the muscles in the center. Slowly bring to the right side and then to left side in a circular way. Do this several times from the right to left side and then do it in a reverse way from the left to right side. You should turn the muscles always with a circular motion slowly. When you advance in the practice you can do it quickly; but you can derive full benefits of this Kriya when you do it very slowly and gradually. This last stage of Nauli will appear like 'churning' when the abdominal muscles are isolated and rotated from side to side.

Beginners will feel slight pain of abdomen in the first two or three attempts. They need not fear and stop the practice. The pain will vanish away in 2 or 3 days. When the advanced Yogic student demonstrates Nauli, the onlookers will be extremely surprised to look at the movements of the abdominal muscles. They will feel as if an engine is working in the abdominal factory.

When beginners want to do Dakshina Nauli, they should slightly bend towards the left side and contract the left muscles. When they want to do Vama Nauli, let them bend a little to the right side. In Madhyama Nauli, push the entire muscles forward by contracting the two sides.

This exercise is not at all possible for those who have a barrel-like belly. When they find it difficult to carry their own belly, they cannot at all dream of getting success in this Kriya. They can also try by gradual slow practice. For getting success, they must exert hard and have rigorous practice for a long time. Those who have a tender body can very easily learn and perform this Kriya in a beautiful and efficient manner.

In the famous Hardwar cosmopolitan platform where Punjabis and Bengali Baboos stroll in the evening with their ladies, on the banks of the Ganges, some persons demonstrate Nauli and various other Asanas and Mudras for the sake of a few pies only. They pass on from one exercise to the other very quickly. You will find the same in Calcutta, Delhi, Bombay, Madras and in all the busy centers. This is only a sort of profession. It is not at all Yoga. It is only a variety of physical feats. From the very condition of their body you will find that they do not possess all the qualifications and aims of a Yogi, They do not even appear physically better, since they are habituated to intoxicant drinks, Ganja, Bhang, etc.

If the Yogic exercises are done in the right way with the right mental attitude, it will surely lead you to spiritual growth. Nauli Kriya eradicates chronic constipation, dyspepsia and all other diseases of the gastro-intestinal system. Nauli helps Sang Pachar and Basti Kriya also. The liver and pancreas are toned. The kidneys and other organs of the abdomen function properly. Nauli is a blessing to humanity. It is a sovereign specific 'uni-all' or an ideal 'pick-me-up.'

5. Trataka

'Trataka' is steady gazing at a particular point or object without winking. Though this is one of the six purificatory exercises, it is mainly intended for developing concentration and mental focusing. It is very useful for the students of Hatha Yoga, Jnana Yoga, Bhakti Yoga and Raja Yoga. There is no other effective method for the control of the mind. Some of the students, who claim that they belong to Jnana Yoga, neglect such important exercises since they are described under Hatha Yogic portions. Sri Ramana Maharshi the famous Jnani of Tiruvannamalai, was doing this exercise. You could have seen it clearly if you had been to his Ashram for his Darshan. While seated on his sofa in his room, he used to gaze on the walls. When he sat on the veranda in an easy chair, he steadily looked at the distant hills or at the sky. This enabled him to keep up a balanced state of mind. Nothing could distract his mind. He was very calm and cool always. He was not at all distracted by any one even though his Bhaktas might be talking and singing by his side.

EXERCISES

(1) Keep the picture of Lord Krishna, Rama, Narayana or Devi in front of you. Look at it steadily without winking. Gaze at the head; then at the body; then at the legs. Repeat the same process again and again. When your mind calms down look at a particular place only. Be steady till tears begin to flow. Then close the eyes and mentally visualize the picture.

(2) Gaze on a black dot on a white wall or draw a black mark on a piece of white paper and hang it on the wall in front of you.

(3) Draw the picture Om (!) on a piece of paper and have it before your seat. Do Trataka on it.

(4) Lie down on an open terrace and gaze at a particular bright star or on the full moon. After some time, you will see different colors of lights. Again some time later,

you will see only a particular color throughout, and all other surrounding stars will disappear. When you gaze at the moon, you will see only a bright moon on a black background. At times you will see a huge mass of light all around you. When gazing becomes more intense, you can also see two or three moons of the same size and at times you cannot see any moon at all even though your eyes may be wide open.

(5) Select at random any place in the open sky in the morning or evening hours and gaze at it steadily. You will get new inspirations.

(6) Look at a mirror and gaze at the pupil of your eye.

(7) Some people do Trataka at the space between the two eyebrows or at the tip of the nose. Even during walking, some persons do Trataka at the tip of the nose.

(8) Advanced students can do Trataka at the inner Chakras, (Padmas). Muladhara, Anahata, Ajna and Sahasrara are the important centers for Trataka.

(9) Keep a ghee-lamp before you and gaze at the flames. Some astral entities give Darshan through the flames.

(10) Very few Yogins do Trataka on the sun. It requires the help of an experienced man by their side. They begin to gaze on the rising sun and after gradual practice they do Trataka on the sun even in the midday. They get some special Siddhis (psychic powers) by this practice. All are not fit for this Sadhana. All the first 9 exercises will suit everyone and they are harmless. The last one, sun gazing should not be attempted until you get the help of an experienced man.

INSTRUCTIONS

When you do the practice in your meditation room, sit in your favorite Asana (posture), Siddhasana or Padmasana. At other times you can do in a standing or sitting posture. Trataka can be profitably done even when you walk. As you walk along the streets, do not look hither and thither. Gaze at the tip of the nose or toes. There are many persons who do not look at the face when they talk to others. They have their own gaze at a particular place and talk. No particular Asana is required for this Sadhana.

When you gaze at a picture, it is Trataka. When you close your eyes and mentally visualize the picture, it is Saguna Dhyana (meditation with form). When you associate the attributes of God such as omnipresence, omnipotence, omniscience, purity, perfection, etc., the name and the form of the object of Trataka will automatically disappear and you will enter into Nirguna Dhyana (abstract meditation).

Do Trataka for two minutes to start with. Then cautiously increase the period. Do not be impatient. Gradual steady practice is required. Gazing at a spot even for three full hours continuously counts for nothing, if the mind is wandering. The mind also must be on the spot. Then only you will advance in this practice and attain many psychic powers.

Those who cannot gaze steadily for a second in spite of several attempts need not worry much. They can close their eyes and gaze at an imaginary spot at the space between the two eyebrows.

Those who have very weak eye-capillaries should do Trataka after closing their eyes on any imaginary spot within or without. Do not tax your eyes by over-practice. When you feel tired, close your eyes and keep your mind on the object of Trataka. When you sit and do Trataka do not shake the body.

Trataka improves eyesight. Many who had some eye-troubles have realized immense benefits by Trataka. Going beyond one's own power and gazing at the sun without any help may produce serious troubles. For gazing on the sun you must have your guide by your side. The Guru will prescribe some oil to rub on your head to avoid such serious troubles and to cool the system. You should apply honey to your eyes at night when you practice sun gazing.

The same object of gazing will appear as something else during the practice. You will have many other visions. Different people have different experiences. You will not even believe certain things when others tell you of their experiences. Trataka alone cannot give you all Siddhis. After the control of the mind, when it becomes steady, you will have to manipulate the mind by prescribed methods for the attainment of powers. Therefore the powers that are obtained by this practice may vary in different persons. It depends upon the further training of the mind, in a particular way.

Young aspirants, who pose as big Yogins, neglect such practices and ask whether this practice is Moksha. Certainly that practice itself is not Moksha. Different practices are for the attainment of Moksha. One can attain the goal by a particular method, others by different methods. Remember this point always. Otherwise you will be neglecting all the methods. You will be misguided and lose the goal if you neglect the Sadhana.

By the practice of Trataka, diseases of the eyes are removed. Eyesight improves. Many have thrown away their spectacles after taking to this practice. Will power is developed. Vikshepa is destroyed. It steadies the mind.

Clairvoyance, thought reading, psychic cure and other Siddhis are obtained very easily.

Once again I will tell you that Bhakti Yoga, Jnana Yoga, Hatha Yoga, Karma Yoga, etc., are not incompatibles like Cocaine and Soda Bicarbonate. They are not antagonistic to each other. Do not neglect this exercise for the mere reason that it comes under Hatha Yoga portions. Even though you may claim to be a student of Jnana Yoga or Bhakti Yoga, you can take to this practice. It is a very effective powerful remedy for a wandering mind. It prepares the mind undoubtedly for perfect Dhyana and Samadhi. This is assuredly a means for the end. You must ascend the Yogic ladder or staircase step by step. Several persons have been benefited by this useful exercise. Why not you, also, dear friend, sincerely attempt to practice this from this moment? I have given you different exercises for Trataka. Select any one of the methods that suits you best and realize the spiritual benefits. Do this for one month regularly and let me know your experiences, benefits and also troubles, if any.

6. Kapalabhati

Kapalabhati is an exercise for the purification of skull and lungs. Though this is one of the Shat-Karmas (six purificatory exercises), yet it is a variety of Pranayama exercises.

Sit in Padmasana or Siddhasana. Keep the hands on the knees. Perform Puraka (inhalation) and Rechaka (exhalation) rapidly. Those who can do Bhastrika Pranayama can easily do this. In Bhastrika there is a Kumbhaka (retention of breath) for a long time at the end of the required rounds. But in Kapalabhati there is no Kumbhaka. Again in Kapalabhati, Puraka is very long and mild, but Rechaka is too quick and forcible. In Bhastrika,

Puraka is done as quickly as Rechaka. This is the only difference between Kapalabhati and Bhastrika. In Kapalabhati, Rechaka should be done forcibly and quickly by contracting the abdominal muscles with backward push. To start with, have only one expulsion per second. In the beginning do 10 expulsions per round. Gradually increase 10 expulsions to each round till you get 120 expulsions for each round.

It cleanses the respiratory system and nasal passages. It removes spasm in bronchial tubes. Consequently Asthma is relieved and cured also in course of time. Consumption is cured by this practice. Impurities of the blood are thrown out. The circulatory and respiratory systems are toned to a considerable degree. Shat-Karmas are intended for the purification of the body. When Nadis are impure Kundalini cannot pass from the Muladhara to Sahasrara Chakra. Purification of Nadis is effected through Pranayama. For Pranayama, you should know well about Prana.

PRANAYAMA

What Is Prana?

Prana is the sum total of all energy that is manifested in the universe. It is the vital force, Sukshma. Breath is the external manifestation of Prana. By exercising control over this gross breath, you can control the subtle Prana inside. Control of Prana means control of mind. Mind cannot operate without the help of Prana. It is the Sukshma Prana that is intimately connected with the mind. Prana is the sum total of all latent forces which are hidden in men and which lie everywhere around us. Heat, light, electricity, magnetism are all the manifestations of Prana. Prana is related to mind; through mind to the will; through will to the individual soul, and through this to the Supreme Being. The seat of Prana is the heart. Prana is one; but it has many functions to do. Hence it assumes five names according to the different functions it performs, viz., Prana, Apana, Samana, Udana and Vyana. According to the different functions they perform, they occupy certain places in the body. The table given in the following pages will give you a clear idea.

Breath directed by thought under the control of the will is a vitalizing, regenerated force which can be utilized consciously for self-development, for healing many incurable diseases and for many other useful purposes. Hatha Yogins consider that Prana Tattva is superior to Manas Tattva (mind), as Prana is present even when mind is absent during deep sleep. Hence Prana plays a more vital part than mind.

If you know how to control the little waves of Prana working through mind, then you will know the secret of subjugating the universal Prana. The Yogin, who becomes an expert in the knowledge of this secret, will have no fear from any power, because he has mastery over all manifestations of power in the Universe. What is commonly known as Power of Personality is nothing more than the natural capacity of a person to wield his Prana. Some people are more powerful in life, more influential and fascinating than others. It is all through this Prana, which the Yogin uses consciously by the command of his will.

Having acquired a thorough knowledge of the seat of Nadis and of the Vayus with their functions, one should begin with the purification of Nadis. A person possessed of Yama and Niyama, avoiding all company, having finished his course of study, delighting in Truth and virtues, having conquered his anger, being engaged in the service of his spiritual instructor and well instructed in all the religious practices, should go to a secluded place for Yoga Abhyasa.

Five Pranas

NAME	COLOR	LOCATION	REGION	FUNCTION	SUB-PRANAS
Prana	Yellow	Anahata Chakra	Chest	Respiration	1. *Naga* does eructation and hiccup.
Apana	Orange red	Muladhara Chakra	Anus	Discharge of urine and feces	2. *Kurma* performs the function of opening the eyes.
Samana	Green	Manipura Chakra	Navel	Digestion	3. *Krikara* induces hunger and thirst.
Udana	Violet blue	Vishuddha Chakra	Throat	Deglutition. Takes the Jiva to Brahman in sleep. Separates the physical body from the astral body at death	4. *Devadatta* does yawning.
Vyana	Rose	Swadhishthana Chakra	Entire body	Circulation of blood	5. *Dhananjaya* causes decomposition of body

Nadi Suddhi (purification of Nadis) is an important matter in the early stage of Yoga. If there are impurities in the Nadis, the ascent of Kundalini in the Sushumna is seriously retarded. Purity in the Nadis facilitates the ascent of Kundalini. Pranayama brings about quick purification of the Nadis. Nadi Suddhi is the basis of Yoga. It is the foundation of Yoga. It is the first part of Yoga.

Just as you can stop all the other wheels of the factory if you can stop the important flywheel of the engine, so also if you can stop the functions of all other organs of the body, you can get control of the subtle, psychic Prana by restraining the breath. That is the reason why Pranayama is prescribed for controlling Prana.

Prana is the over-coat of the mind. If you can control Prana, you can control mind and Veerya also, because Prana, Veerya and mind are under one Sambandha. If you can control mind, breath stops by itself. Prana comes under control. Just as you have a nervous system in the gross physical body, so also there is a nervous system in the astral body. The nervous system of the physical body is the Sthula Prana. The nervous system of the astral body is the Sukshma Prana. There is intimate connection between these two Pranas. There is inter-action between these two Pranas.

By controlling the act of breathing, you can efficiently control all the various functions in the body. You can very easily and quickly control and develop the body, mind and soul. Psychic cure, Telepathy, Television, thought reading and other Siddhis are the effects of the control of Prana. The process by which the Prana is controlled by regulation of breath is termed 'Pranayama'. It is through Pranayama that you can control your circumstances and character and consciously harmonize the universal individual life with the cosmic life.

Pranayama

To suit the different constitutions, temperament and purpose, in Pranayama there are many varieties of exercises, viz., deep breathing exercise, Sukha Purvaka (easy comfortable) Pranayama during walking, Pranayama during meditation, Rhythmical breathing, Suryabheda, Ujjayi, Sitkari, Sitali, Bhastrika, Bhramari, Murchha, Plavini, Kevala Kumbhaka, etc. Of all the above exercises only the last eight are described in the Hatha Yogic texts.

Nadi Suddhi

Before commencing the practice of Pranayama however, you should clean the Nadis. Then only will you derive the maximum benefit from Pranayama. The cleansing of the Nadi (Nadi-Suddhi) is either Samanu or Nirmanu—that is, with or without the use of Bija. According to the first form, the Yogi in Padmasana or Siddhasana offers his prayers to the Guru and meditates on him. Meditating on 'Yang' (y:ú) he does Japa through Ida of the Bija 16 times, Kumbhaka with Japa of the Bija 64 times, and then exhalation through the solar Nadi and Japa of Bija 32 times. Fire is raised from Manipura and united with Prithvi. Then follows inhalation by the solar Nadi with the Vahni Bija 'Rang' (rú) 16 times, Kumbhaka with Japa of the Bija 64 times, followed by exhalation through the lunar Nadi and Japa of the Bija 32 times. He then meditates on the lunar brilliance, gazing at the tip of the nose, and inhales by Ida with Japa of the Bija 'Thang' (Yú) 16 times. Kumbhaka is done with the Bija 'Vang' (v:ú) 64 times. He thinks himself as flooded by nectar, and considers that the Nadis have been washed. He exhales by Pingala with Japa of the Bija 'Lang' (l:ú) 32 times and considers himself thereby as strengthened.

Now I will tell you a few important exercises only, that are useful in awakening the Kundalini.

1. Sukha Purvaka

(Easy Comfortable Pranayama)

Sit in Padmasana or Siddhasana. Close the right nostril with your right thumb. Inhale (Puraka) through the left nostril till you count 3 Oms slowly. Imagine that you are drawing the Prana along with the atmospheric air. In course of practice, you will actually feel that you are drawing Prana. Then close the left nostril also with the little and ring fingers of your right hand. Retain the breath till you count 12 Oms. Send the current down to the Muladhara Chakra. Feel that the nerve-current is striking against the Muladhara Chakra and awakening Kundalini. Remove the right thumb and exhale through the right nostril till you count 6 Oms. Again inhale through the right nostril, retain and exhale through the left nostril as stated above. All the above six processes constitute one Pranayama. To start with do 6 Pranayamas in the morning and 6 in the evening. Gradually increase it to 20 Pranayamas for each sitting. The ratio of inhalation, retention and exhalation is 1:4:2. You should gradually increase the period of Kumbhaka.

Be careful in doing the Kumbhaka as long as you can comfortably do. Do not be in a hurry. Be patient. Contract the anus and do Mula Bandha also. Concentrate on the Chakra and meditate on Kundalini. This is the most important portion of this exercise. In this Pranayama, deep concentration plays a vital part in awakening Kundalini. Kundalini will be awakened quickly if the degree of concentration is intense and if practiced regularly.

This exercise removes all diseases, purifies the Nadis, steadies the wandering mind, improves digestion and circulation, helps Brahmacharya, and awakens Kundalini. All the impurities of the body are thrown out.

2. Bhastrika

Rapid succession of forcible expulsions is a characteristic feature of this exercise. 'Bhastrika' means 'bellows' in Sanskrit. Just as a blacksmith blows his bellows rapidly, so also you should inhale and exhale rapidly. Sit in your favorite Asana. Close the mouth. Inhale and exhale quickly 20 times like the bellows. Constantly dilate and contract the chest as you inhale and exhale. When you practice the Pranayama a hissing sound is produced. You should start with forcible expulsions of breath following one another in rapid succession. After 20 such expulsions, make a deep inhalation and retain the breath as long as you can comfortably do and then slowly exhale. This is one round of Bhastrika.

Begin with 10 expulsions for a round and increase it gradually to 20 or 25 for a round. The period of Kumbhaka also should be gradually and cautiously increased. Rest a while after one round is over and again begin the next round. Do 3 rounds in the beginning and after due practice, do 20 rounds in the morning and 20 in the evening.

Advanced students do this Pranayama after partial closing of the glottis. They do not make a powerful noise like the beginners. They can do it even in a standing posture.

Bhastrika removes inflammation of the throat, increases the gastric fire, destroys phlegm and all diseases of the nose and lungs, eradicates Asthma, consumption and other diseases which arise from the excess of wind, bile and phlegm. It gives warmth to the body. It is the most effective of all Pranayama exercises. It enables Prana to break through the three Granthis. All the other benefits of Sukha Purvaka Pranayama are obtained in this exercise also.

3. Suryabheda

Sit on Padmasana or Siddhasana. Close the eyes. Keep the left nostril closed with your right ring and little fingers. Slowly inhale without making any sound as long as you can do it comfortably through the right nostril. Then close the right nostril with your right thumb and retain the breath by firmly pressing the chin against the chest (Jalandhara Bandha). Hold the breath till perspiration oozes from the roots of the hair (hair follicles). This point cannot be reached at the very outset. You will have to increase the period of Kumbhaka gradually. This is the limit of the sphere of practice of Suryabheda Kumbhaka. Release the Jalandhara Bandha. Then exhale very slowly without making any sound through the left nostril with the thumb closing the right nostril.

Kumbhakah suryabhedastu
jara-mrityu-vinasakah,
Bodhayet kundalim saktim
dehagnim cha vivardhayet

"The practice of Suryabheda Kumbhaka destroys decay and death and awakens Kundalini."

This Pranayama should again and again be performed, as it purifies the brain and destroys the intestinal worms. It removes the four kinds of evils caused by Vayu and cures Vata (rheumatism). It cures rhinitis and various sorts of neuralgia. The worms that are found in the frontal sinuses are also destroyed.

4. Ujjayi

Sit in your usual Asana. Close the mouth. Inhale slowly through both the nostrils in a smooth, uniform manner.

Retain the breath as long as you can do it comfortably and then exhale slowly through the left nostril by closing the right nostril with your right thumb. Expand the chest when you inhale. During inhalation a peculiar sound is produced owing to the partial closing of glottis. The sound produced during inhalation should be of a mild and uniform pitch. It should be continuous also. This Kumbhaka may be practiced even when walking or standing. Instead of exhaling through the left nostril, you can exhale slowly through both nostrils.

This removes the heat in the head. The practitioner becomes very beautiful. The gastric fire is increased. It removes phlegm in the throat. Asthma, consumption and all sorts of pulmonary diseases are cured. All diseases that arise from deficient inhalation of oxygen and diseases of the heart are cured. Ujjayi Pranayama accomplishes all works. Diseases of phlegm, nerves, enlargement of spleen, dyspepsia, dysentery, consumption, cough or fever never attack the practitioner. Perform Ujjayi to destroy decay and death.

5. Plavini

Practice of this Pranayama demands skill on the part of the students. He who practices this Plavini can do Jalastambha and float on water for any length of time, Mr. 'S', a Yogic student, can float on water for twelve hours at a stretch. He who practices this Plavini Kumbhaka can live on air and dispense with food for some days. The student actually drinks air slowly like water and sends it to the stomach. The stomach gets bloated a bit. If you tap the stomach when it is filled with air, you will get a peculiar tympanic (air) sound. Gradual practice is necessary. The help of one, who is well versed in this Pranayama, is necessary. The student can fill up the stomach with air by gradual belching. After the practice, the air should be completely taken out. It is done by Uddiyana Bandha and hiccough.

6. Pranic Healing

Those who practice Pranayama can impart their Prana for healing morbid diseases. They can also recharge themselves with Prana in no time by practicing Kumbhaka.

Never think that you will be depleted of your Prana by distributing it to others. The more you will give, the more it will flow to you from the cosmic source (Hiranyagarbha). That is the law of Nature. Do not become a niggard. If there is a rheumatic patient, gently shampoo his legs with your hands. When you do shampooing (massage), do Kumbhaka and imagine that the Prana is flowing from your hands towards your patient. Connect yourself with Hiranyagarbha or the cosmic Prana and imagine that the cosmic energy is flowing through your hands towards the patient. The patient will at once feel warmth, relief and strength. You can cure headache, intestinal colic or any other disease by massage and by your magnetic touch. When you massage the liver, spleen, stomach or any other portion or organ of the body you can speak to the cells and give them orders: —"O cells! Discharge your functions properly. I command you to do so." They will obey your orders. They too have got subconscious intelligence. Repeat your Mantra when you pass your Prana to others. Try a few cases. You will gain competence. You can cure scorpion-sting also. Gently shampoo the leg and bring the poison down.

You can have extraordinary power of concentration, strong will and a perfectly healthy, strong body by practicing Pranayama regularly. You will have to direct the Prana consciously to unhealthy parts of the body. Suppose you have a sluggish liver. Sit on Padmasana. Close your eyes. Do Sukha Purvaka Pranayama. Direct the Prana to the region of the liver. Concentrate your mind there. Fix your attention to that area. Imagine that Prana is interpenetrating all the tissues and the cells of the lobes of the liver and doing its curative, regenerating and constructive work there. Faith, imagination, attention and interest play a very important part in curing diseases by taking Prana to the diseased areas. During exhalation imagine that the morbid impurities of the liver are thrown out. Repeat this process 12 times in the morning and 12 times in the evening. Sluggishness of liver will vanish in a few days. This is a drugless treatment. This is nature-cure. You can take the Prana to any part of the body during the Pranayama and cure any kind of disease, be it acute or chronic. Try once or twice in healing yourself. Your convictions will grow stronger. Why do you cry like the lady who is crying for ghee when she has butter in her hand, when you have a cheap, potent, easily available remedy or agent 'Prana' at your command at all times! Use it judiciously. When you advance in your concentration and practice, you can cure many diseases by mere touch. In the advanced stages, many diseases are cured by mere will.

7. Distant Healing

This is known as "absent treatment" also. You can transmit Prana through space to your friend who is living at a distance. He should have a receptive mental attitude. You must feel yourself *en rapport* (in direct relation and in sympathy) with the people whom you heal with this Distant Healing method.

You can fix hours of appointment with them through correspondence. You can write to them: "Get ready at 8 p.m. Have a receptive mental attitude. Lie down in an easy chair. Close your eyes. I shall transmit my Prana". Say mentally to the patient, 'I am transmitting a supply of Prana (vital force)'. Do Kumbhaka when you send the Prana. Practice rhythmical breathing also. Have a mental image that the Prana is leaving your mind, passing through space, and is entering the system of the patient. The Prana travels unseen like the wireless (radio) waves and flashes like lightning across space. The Prana that is colored by the thought of the healer is projected outside. You can recharge yourself with Prana by practicing Kumbhaka. This requires long, steady and regular practice.

Importance Of Pranayama

Tamas and Rajas constitute the covering or veil. This veil is removed by the practice of Pranayama. After the veil is removed, the real nature of the soul is realized. The Chitta is by itself made up of Sattvic particles, but Rajas and Tamas envelop it, just as the fire is enveloped by smoke. There is no purificatory action greater than Pranayama. Pranayama gives purity, and the light of knowledge shines. The Karma of the Yogi, which covers up the discriminative knowledge, is annihilated by the practice of Pranayama. By the magic panorama of desire, the essence, which is luminous by nature, is covered up and the Jiva or individual soul is directed towards vice. This Karma of the Yogi, which covers up the Light and binds him to repeated births, becomes attenuated by the practice of Pranayama every moment and is destroyed eventually.

Dharanasu cha Yogyata Manasah: "The mind becomes fit for concentration"—Yoga Sutra (II-53). You will be able to concentrate the mind nicely after this veil of the light has been removed. The mind will be quite steady like the flame in a windless place as the disturbing energy has been removed. The word Pranayama is sometimes used collectively for inhalation, retention and exhalation of breath and sometimes for each of these severally. When the Prana Vayu moves in Akasa Tattva, the breathing will be lessened. At this time it will be easy to stop the breath. The Pranayama will slowly lessen the velocity of the mind. It will induce Vairagya also.

Benefits Of Pranayama

This body becomes lean, strong and healthy. Too much fat is reduced. There is luster in the face. Eyes sparkle like diamonds. The practitioner becomes very handsome. Voice becomes sweet and melodious. The inner Anahata sounds are distinctly heard. The student is free from all sorts of diseases. He gets established in Brahmacharya. Semen gets firm and steady. The Jatharagni (gastric fire) is augmented. The student becomes so perfected in Brahmacharya that his mind will not be shaken even if a fairy tries to embrace him. Appetite becomes keen. Nadis are purified. Vikshepa is removed and the mind becomes one-pointed. Rajas and Tamas are destroyed. The mind is prepared for Dharana and Dhyana. The excretions become scanty. Steady practice arouses the inner spiritual force and brings in spiritual light, happiness and peace of mind. It makes him an Oordhvareto-Yogi. All psychic powers are obtained. Advanced students only will get all the benefits.

Instructions On Pranayama

1. Early morning, answer the calls of nature and sit for the Yogic practices. Practice Pranayama in a dry, welt-ventilated room. Pranayama requires deep concentration and attention. Do not keep anyone by your side.

2. Before you sit for Pranayama practice, thoroughly clean the nostrils. When you finish the practice, take a cup of milk or light tiffin after 10 minutes.

3. Strictly avoid too much talking, eating, sleeping, mixing with friends and exertion. Take a little ghee with rice when you take your meals. This will lubricate the bowels and allow Vayu to move downwards freely.

4. Some people twist the muscles of the face when they do Kumbhaka. It should be avoided. It is also a symptom to indicate that they are going beyond their

capacity. This must be strictly avoided. Such people cannot have a regulated Rechaka and Puraka.

5. Pranayama can also be performed as soon as you get up from bed and just before Japa and meditation. It will make your body light and you will enjoy the meditation. You must have a routine according to your convenience and time.

6. Do not shake the body unnecessarily. By shaking the body often the mind also is disturbed. Do not scratch the body every now and then. The Asana should be steady and as firm as a rock when you do Pranayama, Japa and meditation.

7. In all the exercises, repeat Rama, Siva, Gayatri, or any other Mantra, mere number or any other time-unit according to your inclination. Gayatri or OM is the best for Pranayama. In the beginning you must observe some time-unit for Puraka, Kumbhaka and Rechaka. The time-unit and the proper ratio comes by itself when you do the Puraka, Kumbhaka and Rechaka as long as you can do them comfortably. When you have advanced in the practice, you need not count or keep any unit. You will be naturally established in the normal ratio through force of habit.

8. For some days in the beginning you must count the number and see how you progress. In the advanced stages, you need not distract the mind in counting. The lungs will tell you when you have finished the required number.

9. Do not perform the Pranayama till you are fatigued. There must be always joy and exhilaration of spirit during and after the practice. You should come out of the practice fully invigorated and refreshed. Do not bind yourself by too many rules (Niyamas).

10. Do not take bath immediately after Pranayama is over. Take rest for half an hour. If you get perspiration

during the practice, do not wipe it with a towel. Rub it with your hand. Do not expose the body to the chill draughts of air when you perspire.

11. Always inhale and exhale very slowly. Do not make any sound. In Pranayamas like Bhastrika and Kapalabhati, you can produce a mild or the lowest possible sound.

12. You should not expect the benefits after doing it for 2 or 3 minutes only for a day or two. At least you must have 15 minutes' daily practice in the beginning regularly for days together. There will be no use if you jump from one exercise to another every day.

13. Patanjali does not lay much stress on the practice of different kinds of Pranayama. He mentions: "Exhale slowly, then inhale and retain the breath. You will get a steady and calm mind." It was only the Hatha Yogins who developed Pranayama as a science and who have mentioned various exercises to suit different persons.

14. A neophyte should do Puraka and Rechaka only without any Kumbhaka for some days. Take a long time to do Rechaka. The proportion for Puraka and Rechaka is 1:2.

15. "Pranayama in its popular and preparatory form may be practiced by everyone in any posture whatsoever, sitting or walking; and yet it is sure to show its benefits. For those who practice it in accordance with the prescribed methods, fructification will be rapid."

16. Gradually increase the period of Kumbhaka. Retain for 4 seconds in the first week, for 8 seconds in the second week and for 12 seconds in the third week and so on till you are able to retain the breath to your full capacity.

17. You must so nicely adjust the Puraka, Kumbhaka and Rechaka that you should not experience the feeling of suffocation or discomfort at any stage of Pranayama. You should never feel the necessity of catching hold of a few

normal breaths between any two successive rounds. The duration of Puraka, Kumbhaka and Rechaka must be properly adjusted. Exercise due care and attention. Matters will turn out to be successful and easy.

18. You must not unnecessarily prolong the period of exhalation. If you prolong the time of Rechaka, the following inhalation will be done in a hurried manner and the rhythm will be disturbed. You must so carefully regulate the Puraka, Kumbhaka and Rechaka that you must be able to do with absolute comfort and care, not only of one Pranayama but also the full course or required rounds of Pranayama. I have to repeat this often. Experience and practice will make one perfect. Be steady. Another important factor is that you must have efficient control over the lungs at the end of Kumbhaka to enable you to do the Rechaka smoothly and in proportion with the Puraka.

ASANAS

Importance Of Asanas

Four Asanas are prescribed for the purpose of Japa and meditation. They are Padmasana, Siddhasana, Svastikasana and Sukhasana. You must be able to sit in any one of these four Asanas at a stretch for full three hours without shaking the body. Then only you will get Asana-Jaya, mastery over the Asana. Without securing a steady Asana, you cannot further get on well in meditation. The steadier you are in your Asana, the more you will be able to concentrate and make your mind one-pointed. If you can be steady in the posture even for one hour, you will be able to acquire one-pointed mind and feel thereby infinite peace and Atmic Ananda.

When you sit on the posture, think: "I am as firm as a rock". Give this suggestion to the mind half a dozen times. Then the Asana will become steady soon. You must become as a living statue when you sit for Dhyana. Then only there will be real steadiness in your Asana. In one year by regular practice you will have success and will be able to sit for three hours at a stretch. Start with half an hour and gradually increase the period.

When you sit in the Asana, keep your head, neck and trunk in one straight line. Stick to one Asana and make it quite steady and perfect by repeated attempts. Never change the Asana. Adhere to one tenaciously. Realize the full benefits of one Asana. Asana gives Dridhata (strength). Mudra gives Sthirata (steadiness). Pratyahara gives Dhairya (boldness). Pranayama gives Laghima (lightness). Dhyana gives Pratyakshatva (perception) of Self and Samadhi gives Kaivalya (isolation) which is verily the freedom or final beatitude.

The postures are as many in number as there are number of species of living creatures in this universe. There are 84 lakhs of Asanas described by Lord Siva. Among them 84 are the best and among these, 32 are very useful. There are some Asanas which can be practiced while standing. These are Tadasana, Trikonasana, Garudasana, etc. There are some which can be practiced by sitting, such as Paschimottanasana, Padmasana, etc. Some Asanas are done while lying down. These are Uttanapadasana, Pavanamuktasana, etc. Sirshasana, Vrikshasana, etc., are done with head downwards and legs upwards.

In olden days these Asanas were practiced in Gurukulas and so the people were strong and healthy and had long lives. In schools and colleges these Asanas should be introduced. Ordinary physical exercises develop the superficial muscles of the body only. One can become a

Sandow with a beautiful physique by the physical exercises. But Asanas are intended for physical and spiritual development.

Detailed instructions regarding the technique of 94 Asanas are given in my book 'Yoga Asanas' with illustrations. Here I will mention only a few of the Asanas that are useful for concentration, meditation and for awakening the Kundalini.

1. Padmasana (Lotus Pose)

Amongst the four poses prescribed for Japa and Dhyana, Padmasana comes foremost. It is the best Asana for contemplation. Rishis like Gheranda, Sandilya, speak very highly of this vital Asana. This is highly agreeable for householders. Even ladies can sit in this Asana. Padmasana is suitable for lean persons and for youths as well.

Sit on the ground by spreading the legs forward. Then place the right foot on the left thigh and the left foot on the right thigh. Place the hands on the knee-joints. You can make a fingerlock and keep the locked hands over the left ankle. This is very convenient for some persons. Or you can place the left hand over the left knee and then place the right hand over the right knee with the palm facing upwards and the index finger touching the middle portion of the thumb (Chinmudra).

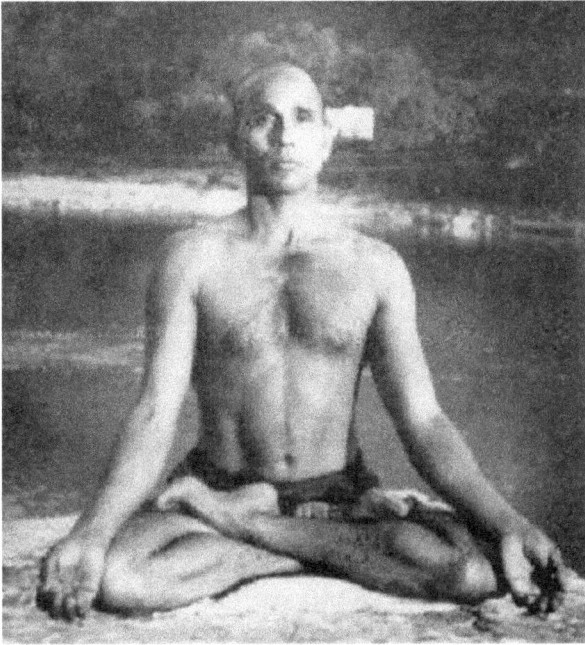

PADMASANA

2. Siddhasana (The Perfect Pose)

Next to Padmasana comes Siddhasana in importance. Some eulogize this Asana as even superior to Padmasana for purposes of Dhyana. If you get mastery over this Asana, you will acquire many Siddhis. Further many Siddhas of yore were practicing it. Hence the name Siddhasana.

Even fatty persons with big thighs can practice this Asana easily. In fact this is better to some persons than Padmasana. Young Brahmacharins who attempt to get established in celibacy should practice this Asana. This Asana is not suitable for ladies.

Place one heel at anus. Keep the other heel on the root of the generative organ. The feet or legs should be so nicely arranged that the ankle-joints should touch each other. Hands can be placed as in Padmasana.

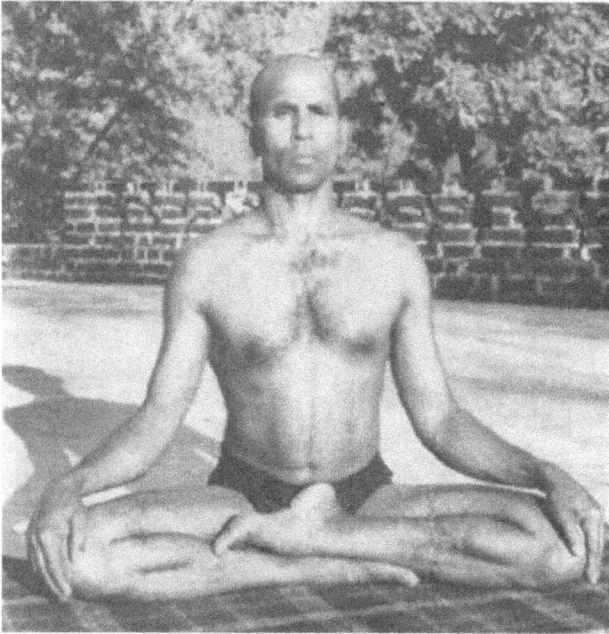

SIDDHASANA

3. Svastikasana (Prosperous Pose)

Svastikasana is sitting at ease with the body erect. Spread the legs forward. Fold the left leg and place the foot near the right thigh muscles. Similarly bend the right leg and push it in the space between the thigh and calf muscles. Now you will find the two feet between the thighs and calves of the legs. This is a very comfortable Asana. Those who find it difficult to do this can sit in Samasana.

Place the left heel at the beginning of right thigh and the right heel at the beginning of the left thigh. Sit at ease. Do not bend either on the left or right. This is called 'Samasana'.

4. Sukhasana

Any easy, comfortable posture for Japa and meditation is Sukhasana; the important point being the head, neck and trunk should be in a line without curve. People who begin Japa and meditation after 30 or 40 years of age generally are not able to sit in Padma, Siddha or Svastikasana for a long time. People sit in any wrong way and they call it 'Sukhasana'. The trouble is even without their knowledge the backbone forms a curve in a few minutes. Now I will describe to you a nice Sukhasana whereby old persons can sit and meditate for a long time. Young persons should not try this. This is specially designed to suit old people who are unable to sit in Padmasana or Siddhasana in spite of repeated attempts.

Take a cloth 5 cubits long. Fold it nicely length-wise till the width becomes half a cubit. Sit in your usual way keeping the feet below your thighs. Raise the two knees to the level of your chest till you get a space of 8 or 10 inches between the knees. Now take the folded cloth. Keep one end near the left side, touching the right knee, come to the starting point. Then make a knot of the two ends. Keep your palms face to face and place them on the support of the cloth between the knees. In this Asana the hands, legs and backbone are supported. Hence you will never feel tired. If you cannot do any other Asana sit at least in this Asana and do Japa and meditation for a long time. You can also have Svadhyaya (study of religious books) in this Asana.

5. Sirshasana (Topsy Turvy Pose)

Spread a four-folded blanket. Sit on the two knees. Make a finger-lock by interweaving the fingers. Place it on the ground up to the elbow. Now keep the top of your head on this finger-lock or between the two hands. Slowly raise the legs till they become vertical. Stand for five seconds in the beginning and gradually increase the period by 15 seconds each week to 20 minutes or half an hour. Then very slowly, bring it down. Strong people will be able to keep the Asana for half an hour within 2 or 3 months. Do it slowly. There is no harm. If you have time, do twice daily both morning and evening. Perform this Asana very, very slowly, to avoid jerks. While standing on the head, breathe slowly through the nose and never through the mouth.

You can place the hands on the ground one on each side of the head. You will find this easy to practice, if you are fat. If you have learnt balancing, you can take to the finger-lock method. This Asana is nothing for those who can balance on parallel bars or on the ground. Ask your friend to assist you to keep the legs steady while practicing or get the help of a wall.

In the beginning some persons may have a novel sensation during practice but this vanishes soon. It brings joy and glee. After the exercise is over take a little rest for five minutes and then take a cup of milk. There are people who are doing this Asana for two or three hours at one stroke.

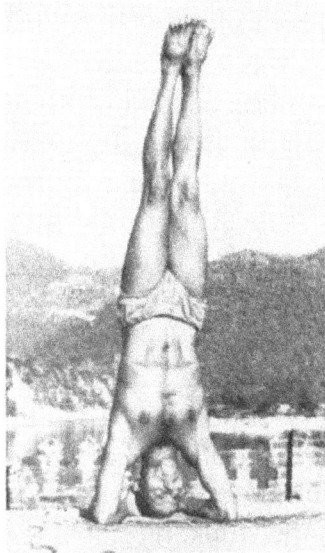

SIRSHASANA

BENEFITS

This is very useful in keeping up Brahmacharya. It makes you Oordhvaretas. The seminal energy is transmuted into spiritual energy, Ojas-Shakti. This is also called sex-sublimation. You will not have wet dreams, Spermatorrhea. In an Oordhvareto-Yogi the seminal energy flows upwards into the brain for being stored up as spiritual force which is used for contemplative purposes (Dhyana). When you do this Asana, imagine that the seminal energy is being converted into Ojas and is passing along the spinal column into the brain for storage.

Sirshasana is really a blessing and a nectar. Words will fail to adequately describe its beneficial results and effects. In this Asana alone, the brain can draw plenty of Prana and blood. Memory increases admirably. Lawyers, occultists and thinkers will highly appreciate this Asana. This leads to natural Pranayama and Samadhi by itself. No other effort is necessary. If you watch the breath, you will notice it becoming finer and finer. In the beginning of practice there will be a slight difficulty in breathing. As you advance in practice, this vanishes entirely. You will find real pleasure and exhilaration of spirit in this Asana.

Great benefit is derived by sitting for meditation after Sirshasana. You can hear Anahata sound quite distinctly. Young, robust persons should perform this Asana. Householders who practice this should not have frequent sexual intercourse.

6. Sarvangasana (All-Members Pose)

This is a mysterious Asana which gives wonderful benefits. Spread a thick blanket on the floor and practice this Asana on the blanket. Lie on the back quite flat. Slowly raise the legs. Lift the trunk, hips, and legs quite vertically. Support the back with the two hands, one on either side. Rest the elbows on the ground. Press the chin against the chest (Jalandhara Bandha). Allow the back-shoulder portion and neck to touch the ground closely. Do not allow the body to shake or move to and fro. Keep the legs straight. When the Asana is over, bring the legs down very, very slowly with elegance and not with any jerks. In this Asana the whole weight of the body is thrown on the shoulders. You really stand on the shoulders with the help and support of the elbows. Concentrate on the Thyroid gland which lies on the front lower part of the neck. Retain the breath as long as you can do with comfort, and slowly exhale through the nose.

You can do this Asana twice daily, morning and evening. This should immediately be followed by Matsyasana (fish-posture). This will relieve pains in the back part of the neck and intensify the usefulness of Sarvangasana. Stand on the Asana for two minutes and gradually increase the period to half an hour.

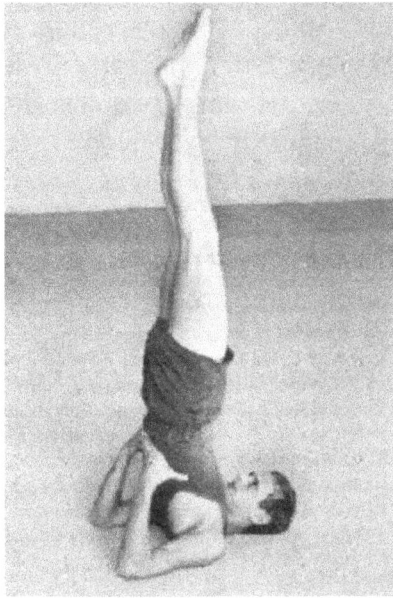

SARVANGASANA

BENEFITS

This is a *panacea*, a cure-all, and a sovereign specific for all diseases. It brightens the psychic faculties and awakens Kundalini Sakti, removes all sorts of diseases of intestine and stomach, and augments the mental power.

It supplies a large quantity of blood to the roots of spinal nerves. It is this Asana which centralizes the blood in the spinal column and nourishes it beautifully. But for this Asana there is no scope for these nerve-roots to draw sufficient blood-supply. It keeps the spine quite elastic. Elasticity of the spine means everlasting youth. It stimulates you in your work. It prevents the spine from early ossification (hardening). So you will preserve and retain your youth for a long time. It helps a lot in maintaining Brahmacharya. Like Sirshasana, it makes you an Oordhvaretas. It checks wet dreams effectively. It rejuvenates those who have lost their potency. It acts as a powerful blood-tonic and purifier. It tones the nerves and awakens Kundalini. Spinal column is rendered very soft and elastic. This Asana prevents the early ossification of the vertebral bones. Ossification is quick degeneration of bones. Old age manifests quickly on account of early ossification. The bones become hard and brittle in the degenerative process. He who practices Sarvangasana is very nimble, agile, full of energy. The muscles of the back are alternately contracted, relaxed and then pulled and stretched. Hence they draw a good supply of blood by these various movements and are well nourished. Various sorts of myalgia (muscular rheumatism), lumbago, sprain, neuralgia, etc., are cured by this Asana.

The vertebral column becomes as soft and elastic as rubber. It is twisted and rolled as it were like a piece of canvas sheet. A man who practices this Asana can never become lazy even a bit. He is a two-legged talking squirrel. The vertebral column is a very important structure. It supports the whole body. It contains the spinal cord, spinal nerve and sympathetic system. In Hatha Yoga the spine is termed as Meru Danda. Therefore you must keep it healthy, strong and elastic. The muscles of the abdomen, the rectic muscles and the muscles of the thigh are also toned and nourished well. Obesity or corpulence and habitual chronic constipation, Gulma, congestion and enlargement of the liver and spleen are cured by this Asana.

7. Matsyasana (Fish Posture)

This Asana will help one to float on water easily with Plavini Pranayama. Therefore it is called fish-pose, Matsyasana. Spread a blanket and sit on Padmasana by keeping the right foot over the left thigh and the left over right thigh. Then lie flat on the back. Hold the head by the two elbows. This is one variety.

Stretch the head back, so that the top of your head rests on the ground firmly on one side and the buttocks only on the other, thus making a bridge or an arch of the trunk. Place the hands on the thighs or catch the toes with the hands. You will have to give a good twisting to the back. This variety is more efficacious than the former one. The benefits that you derive from this variety are a hundred times more than what you get in the previous variety.

Those fatty persons with thick calves, who find it difficult to have Padmasana (foot-lock), may simply sit in the ordinary way and then practice this Asana. Practice the Padmasana first. Make it firm, easy and steady. Then take Matsyasana. Do this Asana for 10 seconds in the beginning and increase it to 10 minutes.

When you have finished the Asana, slowly release the head with the help of hands and get up. Then unlock the Padmasana.

You must practice this Asana soon after Sarvangasana. It will relieve stiffness of the neck and all crampy conditions of the cervical region caused by long practice of Sarvangasana. This gives natural massage or shampooing to the congested parts of the neck and shoulders. Further it affords the maximum benefits of Sarvangasana. It is a complimentary Asana of Sarvangasana. Rather it supplements Sarvangasana. As the larynx or wind-box and trachea (wind-pipe) are thrown open widely, this Asana helps deep breathing.

Matsyasana is the destroyer of many diseases. It removes constipation. It brings down the accumulated fecal matter to the rectum. It is useful in asthma, consumption, chronic bronchitis, etc., on account of the deep breathing.

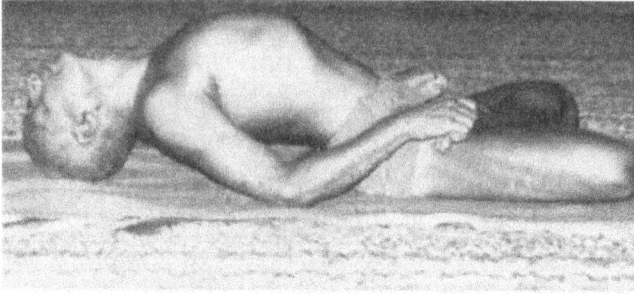

MATSYASANA

8. Paschimottanasana

Sit on the ground and stretch the legs stiff like a stick. Catch the toes with the thumb and index and middle fingers. While catching, you have to bend the trunk forwards. Fatty persons will find it rather difficult to bend. Exhale. Slowly bend without jerks till your forehead touches your knees. You can keep the face even between the knees. When you bend down, draw the belly back. This facilitates the bending forward. Bend slowly by gradual degrees. Take your own time. There is no hurry. When you bend down, bend the head between the hands. Retain it on a level with them. Young persons with elastic spine can touch the knees with the forehead even in their very first attempt. In the case of grown-up persons with rigid spinal column, it will take a fortnight or a month for complete success in the posture. Retain the breath till you take the forehead back, to its original position, till you sit straight again. Then breathe.

Retain the pose for 5 seconds. Then gradually increase the period to 10 minutes.

Those who find it difficult to do the full Paschimottanasana, can do half pose with one leg and one hand and then with the other leg and hand. They will find this easier. After some days when the spine has become more elastic, they can have recourse to the full pose. You will have to use common sense while practicing Yogasanas.

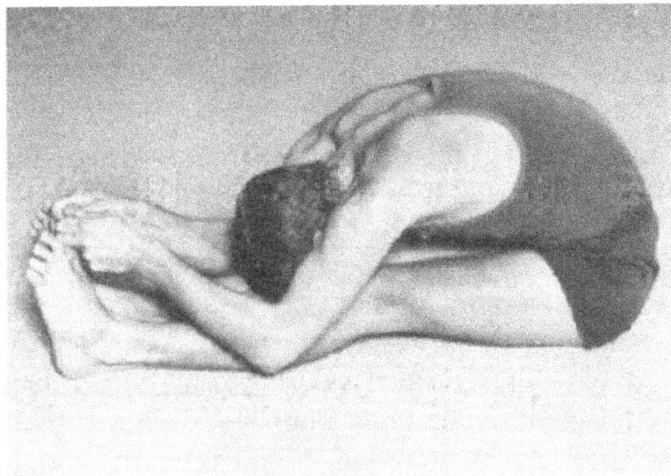

PASCHIMOTTANASANA

BENEFITS

This is an excellent Asana. It makes the breath flow through the Brahma Nadi and Sushumna, and rouses the gastric fire. It reduces fat in the abdomen and makes the loins lean. This Asana is a specific for corpulence or obesity. It brings about reduction of spleen and liver in cases of enlargement of spleen. What Sarvangasana is for the stimulation of endocrine glands, so is Paschimottanasana for the stimulation of abdominal viscera, such as kidneys, liver, pancreas, etc. This Asana relieves constipation, removes sluggishness of liver, dyspepsia, belching and gastritis. Lumbago and all sorts of myalgia of the back muscles are cured. This Asana cures piles and diabetes also. The muscles of the abdomen, the solar plexus, the epigastric plexus, bladder prostate, lumbar nerves, sympathetic cord are all toned up and kept in a healthy, sound condition.

9. Mayurasana (Peacock Pose)

This is more difficult than Sarvangasana. This demands good physical strength.

Kneel on the ground. Sit on the toes. Raise the heels up. Join the two forearms together. Place the palms of the two hands on the ground. The two little fingers must be in close touch. They project towards the feet. Now you have got steady and firm forearms for supporting the whole body in the ensuing elevation of the trunk and legs. Now bring down the abdomen slowly against the conjoined elbows. Support your body upon your elbows that are pressed now against the navel or umbilicus. This is the first stage. Stretch your legs and raise the feet stiff and straight on a level with the head. This is second stage.

Neophytes (beginners) find it difficult to keep up the balance as soon as they raise the feet from the ground. Place a cushion in front. Sometimes you will have a fall forwards and you may hurt your nose slightly. Try to slip on the sides when you cannot keep up the balance. If you find it difficult to stretch the two legs backwards at one stroke, slowly stretch one leg first and then the other. If you adopt the device of leaning the body forwards and head downwards the feet will by themselves leave the ground and you can stretch them quite easily. When the Asana is in full manifestation the head, trunk, buttocks, thighs, legs and feet will be in one straight line and parallel to the ground. This posture is very beautiful to look at.

Beginners can practice this Asana by holding on to a table. They will find it easy to practice this. If you understand the technique of this Asana and if you use your common sense you can do it easily and can keep up the balance without much difficulty. Fatty people have frequent nasty falls, slips and doublings and they excite much laughter amongst the onlookers. Do not bend the legs when you stretch them.

Practice this Asana from 5 to 20 seconds. Those who have good physical strength can do it for 2 or 3 minutes. Retain the breath when you raise the body. It will give you immense strength. When you finish the Asana, exhale slowly.

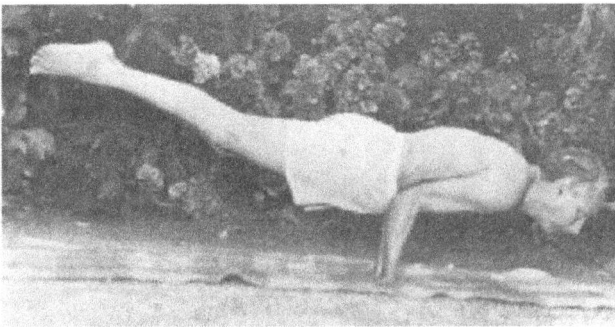

MAYURASANA

BENEFITS

This is a wonderful Asana for improving digestion. It destroys the effects of unwholesome food, and increases the digestive power. It cures dyspepsia and diseases of the stomach like Gulma (chronic gastritis), and reduces spleenic and liver enlargements by increasing the intra-abdominal pressure. The whole abdominal organs are properly toned and stimulated well by the increase of intra-abdominal pressure. Sluggishness of liver or hepatic torpidity disappears. It tones the bowels and removes constipation (ordinary, chronic and habitual). It awakens Kundalini.

10. Ardha Matsyendrasana

Paschimottanasana and Halasana bend the spine forwards. Dhanur, Bhujanga and Salabha Asanas are counter-poses to bend the spine backwards. This is not sufficient. It must be twisted and bent from side to side also (lateral movements). Then only perfect elasticity of the spinal column can be ensured. The Matsyendrasana serves this purpose well in giving a lateral twist to the spinal column.

Place the left heel near the anus and below the scrotum. It can touch the perennial space. Do not allow the heel to move from this space. Bend the knee and place the right ankle at the root of the left thigh and rest the right foot well on the ground close to the left hip joint. Place the left *axilla* or armpit over the top of the vertically bent right knee. Push the knee now a little to the back so that it touches the back part of the *axilla*. Catch hold of the left foot with left palm. Then applying pressure at the left shoulder-joint slowly twist the spine and turn to the extreme right. Turn the face also to the right as much as you can do. Bring it in a line with the right shoulder. Swing round the right arm towards the back. Catch hold of the left thigh with the right hand. Retain the pose from 5 to 15 seconds. Keep the vertebral column erect. Do not bend. Similarly you can twist the spine to the left side.

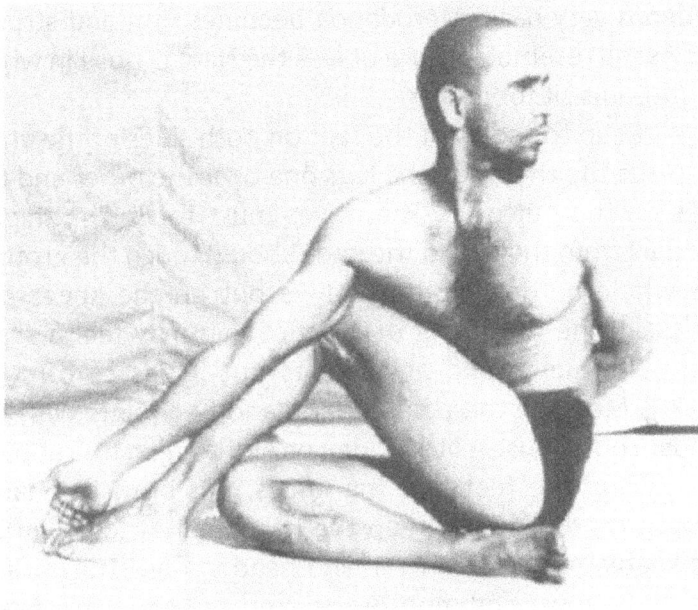

ARDHA MATSYENDRASANA

BENEFITS

This Asana increases appetite by increasing the digestive fire. It destroys terrible diseases. It rouses Kundalini and makes the moon-flow, Chandranadi, steady. Above the root of the palate the moon is said to be located. It drops the cool ambrosial nectar, which is wasted by mixing with gastric fire. But this Asana prevents it.

It keeps the spine elastic and gives a good massage to the abdominal organs. Lumbago and all sorts of muscular rheumatism of the back-muscles are cured. The spinal nerve-roots and sympathetic system are toned. They draw a good supply of blood. This Asana is an adjunct to Paschimottanasana.

11. Vajrasana (The Adamantine Pose)

Those who sit in this Asana have a quite steady and firm pose. They cannot be easily shaken. The knees are rendered very hard. Merudanda becomes firm and strong. This Asana resembles more or less the Namaz pose in which the Muslims sit for prayer.

Keep the soles of the feet on both sides of the anus, i.e., place the thighs on the legs one over the other and the soles on the buttocks. The calves must touch the thighs. The part from the toe to the knee should touch the ground. The whole burden of the body is put on the knees and ankles. In the beginning of practice you may feel a slight pain in the knee and ankle-joints but it passes off very quickly. Massage the painful parts and two joints with the hands. You can use a little Iodex or Amrutanjan for rubbing. After fixing the feet and the knees, put both the hands straight on the knees. Keep the knees quite close. Sit like this keeping the trunk, neck and head in one straight line. This is the most common Asana. You can sit in this Asana for a very long time comfortably. Yogins generally sit in this Asana.

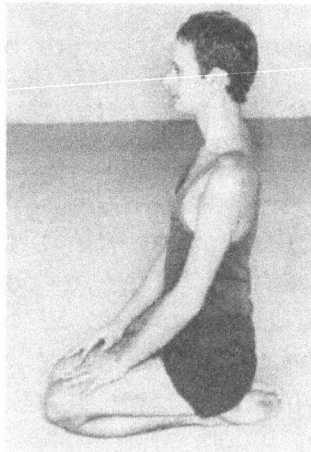

VAJRASANA

BENEFITS

If you sit in this Asana for fifteen minutes immediately after food, the food will be digested well.

Dyspeptics will derive much benefit. The Nadis, nerves and muscles of the legs and thighs are strengthened. Myalgia in the knees, legs, toes and thighs disappears. Sciatica vanishes. Flatulence is removed. Stomach exercises a stimulating, beneficial influence on Kanda, the most vital part from which all the Nadis spring.

12. Urdhva Padmasana (Above Lotus Pose)

Perform Sirshasana. Slowly bend the right leg and keep it on the left thigh and keep the left leg on the right thigh. You must do this very carefully and slowly. If you can stand in Sirshasana for more than 10 or 15 minutes, then you can attempt this. Otherwise you will have a fall and injure your legs. A gymnast, who can balance on the parallel bars on the ground, can do this. The benefits of Sirshasana can be realized from this Asana.

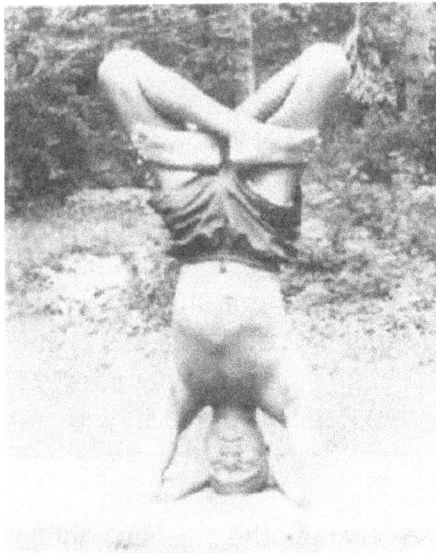

URDHVA PADMASANA

Instructions On Asanas

1. Asana is the first Anga of the Ashtanga Yoga. When you are established in Asana, then only you will derive the benefits of Pranayama.

2. Spread a blanket on the floor and practice the Asanas over the blanket. Use a pillow or four-folded blanket for practicing Sirshasana and its varieties.

3. Wear a Langotee or Kowpeen when you practice Asanas. You can have a banian on the body.

4. Do not wear spectacles when you do Asanas. They may be broken or they will injure your eyes.

5. Those who practice Sirshasana, etc., for a long time, should take light tiffin or a cup of milk after finishing the Asanas.

6. Be regular in the practice. Those who practice by fits and starts will not derive any benefit.

7. Asana should be done on empty stomach in the morning or at least three hours after food. Morning time is best for doing Asanas.

8. If the foundation of a building is not properly laid, the superstructure will fall down in no time, even so if a Yogic student has not gained mastery over the Asanas, he cannot successfully proceed in his higher courses of Yogic practices.

9. Japa and Pranayama should go hand in hand with Yoga Asanas. Then only it becomes real Yoga.

10. In the beginning you cannot perform some of the Asanas perfectly. Regular practice will give perfection. Patience and perseverance, earnestness and sincerity are needed.

11. Never change the Asanas. Adhere to one set tenaciously. If you do one set of Asanas today and some other tomorrow and so on, you cannot derive any benefit.

12. The more steady you are on the Asana the more you will be able to concentrate and make your mind one-

pointed. You cannot get on well in your meditation without having a steady posture.

13. Mild Kumbhaka during the practice of Asanas augments the efficacy of Asanas and give increased power and vitality to the practitioner.

14. Everyone should select a course of a few Asanas to suit his temperament, capacity, convenience, leisure and requirement.

15. If you are careful about your diet, Asanas and meditation, you will have fine, lustrous eyes, fair complexion and peace of mind in a short time. Hatha Yoga ensures beauty, strength and spiritual success to the Yogic students.

16. A man can sit for 10 hours at one stretch motionless on the Asana and yet he may be full of desires. This is a mere physical practice like an acrobatic or circus feat. A man without dosing the eyes, without winking, without turning the eyeballs can practice Tratak for three hours and yet he may be full of desires and egoism. This is also another kind of physical exercise. This has nothing to do with spirituality. People are deceived when they see persons who can do the above practices. Fasting for 40 days is also another kind of training of the physical body.

17. Pranayama with Asanas before starting Japa and meditation is very good and conducive. It removes laziness and drowsiness of the body and mind. It steadies the mind also. It fills the mind with new vigor and peace.

18. Asanas can be practiced on the sandy bed of rivers, open airy places and by seaside also. If you practice them in a room, see that the room is not congested. You should clean it every day.

19. A Vedantin is afraid to do Asanas on the ground that the practice will intensify Dehadhyasa and militate against his practice of Vairagya. I have seen many Vedantins

in a sickly condition with poor physique and dilapidated constitution. They can hardly do any rigid Sadhana. They may utter: "Om Om Om," mechanically through lips only. They have not sufficient strength to raise the Brahmakara Vritti.

20. The body is closely related to the mind. Sickly, weak body is Jada. The body is an important instrument for Self-realization. The instrument must be kept clean, strong and healthy.

MUDRAS AND BANDHAS

Exercises

Mudras and Bandhas are certain postures of the body by which Kundalini is successfully awakened. In Gheranda Samhita, the description of 25 Mudras and Bandhas is given. The following 12 are the most important:
— Many of the above exercises have intimate connection with each other. In one exercise you will have to combine 2 or 3 Bandhas and Mudras. This you will see when you see the description. Many aspirants are not able to find out the exact technique of several Mudras that are described in Hatha Yogic texts, and therefore they could not realize the benefits.

Yogic exercises when practiced regularly in the right way, will surely bestow on you all that you want.

Nasti mudrasamam kinchit
Siddhidam kshitimandale
"There is nothing in this world like Mudras for giving success."

Mudras and Bandhas cure dyspepsia, constipation, piles, cough, asthma, enlargement of spleen, venereal diseases, leprosy and all sorts of incurable diseases. They are the most effective exercises for maintaining Brahmacharya, without which nothing can be made in the spiritual path.

1. Mula Bandha

Press the Yoni with the left heel. Keep the right heel pressed at the space just above the organ of generation. Contract the anus and draw the Apana Vayu upwards. This is called Mula Bandha. The Apana Vayu, which does the function of ejection of excreta, has natural tendency to move downwards. Through the practice of Mula Bandha, the Apana Vayu is made to move upwards by contracting the anus and by forcibly drawing it upwards. The Prana Vayu is united with the Apana and the united Prana-Apana Vayu is made to enter the Sushumna Nadi. Then the Yogi attains perfection in Yoga. Kundalini is awakened. The Yogi drinks the Nectar of Immortality. He enjoys Siva-pada in Sahasrara Chakra. He gets all divine Vibhutis and Aishvarya. When the Apana is united with Prana, Anahata sounds (mystical inner sounds) are heard very distinctly. Prana, Apana, Nada and Bindu unite and the Yogi reaches perfection in Yoga. This highest stage cannot be reached by the first attempt. One should practice this again and again for a long time.

The Siddhi in the practice of Pranayama is attained through the help of Bandhas and Mudras. The practice of Mula Bandha enables one to keep up perfect Brahmacharya, gives Dhatu-Pushti (nerve-vigor), relieves constipation and increases Jatharagni. During the practice of concentration, meditation, Pranayama and all other Yogic Kriyas, Mula Bandha can be combined.

2. Jalandhara Bandha

Contract the throat. Press the chin firmly against the chest. This Bandha is practiced at the end of Puraka and beginning of Kumbhaka. Generally this Bandha is done during Kumbhaka only. The gastric fire, which is situated in the region of Nabhi, consumes the nectar which exudes out of the Sahasrara Chakra through the hole in the palate. This Bandha prevents the nectar being thus consumed.

3. Uddiyana Bandha

The Sanskrit word "Uddiyana" comes from the root 'ut' and 'di' which means to "fly up." When this Bandha is practiced the Prana flies up through the Sushumna Nadi. Hence the significant name.

Empty the lungs by a strong and forcible expiration. The lungs will become completely empty when you exhale forcibly through the mouth. Now contract and draw up the intestines above and below the navel towards the back, so that the abdomen rests against the back of the body high up in the thoracic cavity. This is Uddiyana Bandha. This is practiced at the end of Kumbhaka and beginning of the Rechaka. When you practice this Bandha, the diaphragm, the muscular portion between the thoracic cavity and abdomen, is raised up and the abdominal muscles are drawn backwards. If you bend your trunk forwards, you can easily do this exercise. Uddiyana Bandha is the first stage of Nauli Kriya. You should know Uddiyana Bandha if you want to practice Nauli Kriya. Nauli Kriya is generally done in a standing position. Uddiyana Bandha can be practiced in a sitting or standing posture. When you do it while standing, keep your hands on the thigh as shown in the illustration.

This exercise helps a lot in keeping up Brahmacharya. It imparts beautiful health, strength, vigor and vitality to the practitioner. When it is combined with Nauli Kriya, it serves as a powerful gastro-intestinal tonic. These are the two potent weapons of the Yogin to combat against constipation, weak peristalsis of the intestines and other disorders of the alimentary canal. It is by these two Yogic Kriyas alone, that you can manipulate and massage all the abdominal muscles. For abdominal exercises nothing can compete with Uddiyana Bandha and Nauli. They stand unique and unrivalled amongst all systems of physical exercises. In chronic diseases of stomach and intestines, where drugs of all sorts have failed, Uddiyana and Nauli have effected a rapid, thorough and marvelous cure.

When you practice Pranayama, you can beautifully combine Mula Bandha, Jalandhara Bandha and Uddiyana Bandha. This is Bandha-Traya.

Uddiyana Bandha reduces fat in the belly. In cases where Marienbud reduction pills have failed to reduce fat, Uddiyana Bandha will work wonders. If fatty persons stop taking ghee and reduce the quantity of drinking water, they will be able to do Uddiyana. A trip to Kedar-Badri or Mount Kailas by foot will prepare fatty people for the practice of Uddiyana Bandha.

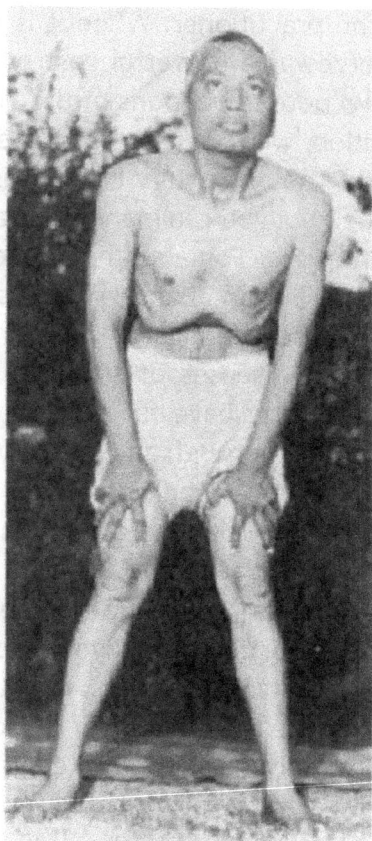

UDDIYANA BANDHA

4. Maha Mudra

This is the most important of all Mudras. Hence it is called 'Maha Mudra.' Press the anus carefully with the left heel. Stretch out the right leg. Catch hold of the toe with the two hands. Inhale and retain the breath. Press the chin against the chest firmly (Jalandhara Bandha). Fix the gaze between the eyebrows (Bhrumadhya Drishti). Retain the posture as long as you can and then exhale slowly. Practice first on the left leg and then on the right leg.

This cures consumption, hemorrhoids or piles, enlargement of spleen, indigestion, Gulma (chronic

156

gastritis), leprosy, constipation, fever and all other diseases. Life is increased. It confers great Siddhis on the practitioners. Generally the Yogi does Maha Mudra, Maha Bandha and Maha Vedha. This is a good combination. Then only maximum benefits are derived. Do like this six times in the morning and evening.

5. Maha Bandha

Maha Mudra is the preliminary exercise for this. Press the anus with the left heel. Place the right foot upon the left thigh. Contract the anus and muscles of the perineum. Draw the Apana Vayu upwards. Draw the breath slowly and retain it by Jalandhara Bandha as long as you can. Then exhale slowly. Practice first on the left side and then on the right side. The Bandha destroys decay and death. The Yogi achieves all his desires and obtains Siddhis.

6. Maha Vedha

Sit in Maha Bandha posture. Draw the breath slowly. Retain the breath. Press the chin against the chest. Place the palms on the ground. Rest the body on the palms. Raise the buttocks slowly and strike them gently against the ground. The Asana must be intact and firm when you raise the buttocks. This Kriya destroys decay and death. The Yogi gets control over the mind and conquers death. There is not much difference between Maha Mudra, Maha Bandha and Maha Vedha. They are something like 3 stages of one exercise.

7. Yoga Mudra

Sit in Padmasana. Place the palms on the heels. Exhale slowly and bend forwards and touch the ground with the forehead. If you retain the pose for a long time, you can breathe as usual. Or come to the former position and inhale. Instead of keeping the hands on the heels, you can take them to the back. Catch hold of the left wrist with your right hand. This pose removes all kinds of disorders of the abdomen.

8. Viparitakarani Mudra

Lie on the ground. Raise the legs up straight. Support the buttocks with the hands. Rest the elbows on the ground. Remain steady. The sun dwells at the root of the navel and the moon at the root of the palate. The process by which the sun is brought upward and the moon is carried downward is called Viparitakarani Mudra. The positions of the sun and the moon are reversed. On the first day do it for a minute. Gradually increase the period to three hours. After six months wrinkles on the face and gray hair disappear. The Yogin who practices this for three hours daily conquers death. As the gastric fire is increased, those who practice this Mudra for a long time should take some light refreshment such as milk, etc., as soon as the Kriya is over. Sirshasana posture also is called Viparitakarani Mudra.

9. Khechari Mudra

'Kha' means Akasa and 'Chari' means to move. The Yogi moves in the Akasa. The tongue and the mind remain in the Akasa. Hence this is known as Khechari Mudra.

A man can perform this Mudra, only if he has undergone the preliminary exercise under the direct guidance of a Guru, who is practicing Khechari Mudra. The preliminary portion of this Mudra is in making the tongue so long that the tip of the tongue might touch the space between the two eyebrows. The Guru will cut the lower tendon of the tongue with a bright, clean knife little by little every week. By sprinkling salt and turmeric powder, the cut edges may not join together again. Cutting the lower tendon of the tongue should be done regularly, once a week, for a period of six months. Rub the tongue with fresh butter and draw it out. Take hold of the tongue with the fingers and move it to and fro. Milking the tongue means taking hold of it and drawing it as the milkman does the udder of a cow during milking. By all these means you can lengthen the tongue to reach the forehead. This is the preliminary portion of Khechari Mudra.

Then turn the tongue upwards and backwards by sitting in Siddhasana so as to touch the palate and close the posterior nasal openings with the reversed tongue and fix the gaze on the space between the two eyebrows. Now leaving the Ida and Pingala, Prana will move in the Sushumna Nadi. The respiration will stop. The tongue is on the mouth of the well of nectar. This is Khechari Mudra.

By the practice of this Mudra the Yogi is free from fainting, hunger, thirst and laziness. He is free from diseases, decay, old age and death. This Mudra makes one an Oordhvaretas. As the body of the Yogi is filled with nectar, he will not die even by virulent poison. This Mudra gives Siddhis to Yogins. Khechari is the best of all Mudras.

10. Vajroli Mudra

This is an important Yogic Kriya in Hatha Yoga. You will have to work hard to get full success in this Kriya. There are very few people who are experts in this act. Yogic students draw water first through a silver-tube (catheter specially made) passed into the urethra 12 inches inside. After due practice they draw milk, then oil, honey, etc. They draw mercury in the end. Later on they can draw these liquids directly through the urethra without the help of the silver-tube. This Kriya is of immense use for keeping up perfect Brahmacharya. On the first day you should send the catheter inside the urethra for one inch only, the second day two inches, third day three inches, and so on. You must gradually practice till you are able to send 12 inches of the catheter inside. The way becomes clear and blowing. Raja Bhartrihari could do this Kriya very dexterously.

Even a drop of semen cannot come out of the Yogi who practices this Mudra. Even if it is discharged, he can draw it back through this Mudra. The Yogi, who draws his semen up and preserves it, conquers death. Good smell emanates from his body.

The late Trilingaswami of Varanasi was an expert in this Kriya. Sri Swami Kuvalayanandaji of Lonavala teaches this Mudra.

Some persons call the Mayurasana Vajroli Mudra. Again Vajroli Mudra is also known as Yoni Mudra. However, the description of Yoni Mudra is given separately.

The object of Vajroli Mudra is to be perfectly established in Brahmacharya. When aspirants practice this Mudra, they unconsciously divert their mind to sexual centers and thereby they cannot get any success. When you see the description of this Mudra, you will clearly understand that strict Brahmacharya is absolutely necessary. For practicing this there is no necessity at all for a woman or for any sexual intercourse. Since the Grihasthas have their wives and because they think that Vajroli Mudra is a device for birth control, they have a keen desire to practice this Mudra. It is all mere foolishness and delusion. They have not understood the technique and object of this important Kriya.

Practice of Mula Bandha, Maha Bandha, Maha Mudra, Asanas, Pranayamas, etc., will naturally enable one to understand and to get success in the practice of Vajroli. This must be done under the direct guidance of a Guru.

11. Shakti Chalana Mudra

Sit in a secluded room in Siddhasana. Draw in the air forcibly and join it with Apana. Do Mula Bandha till the Vayu enters the Sushumna. By retaining the air, the Kundalini, feeling suffocated, awakes and finds its way through Sushumna to Brahmarandhra.

Sit in Siddhasana. Take hold of the foot near the ankle and slowly beat the Kanda with the foot. This is Tadana Kriya. By this method also Kundalini can be awakened. Through the practice of this Mudra one can become a Siddha.

12. Yoni Mudra

Sit in Siddhasana. Close the ears with the two thumbs, eyes with the index fingers, nostrils with the middle fingers, the upper lips with the ring fingers and the lower lips with the little fingers. This is a beautiful pose for doing Japa. Dive deep and meditate on the Shat Chakras and Kundalini. This is not quite easy for all like other Mudras. You have to exert much in getting success in this. You must be perfectly established in Brahmacharya if you want sure success. *"Devanamapi durlabha"*—very difficult to be obtained even by Devas. Therefore realize the importance of this Mudra and practice it very cautiously. Vajroli Mudra also is called Yoni Mudra.

Other Mudras

There are Sambhavi, Manduki, Aswini, Tadagi, Matangini, Bhuchari, Aghori and various other Mudras. Here I have told you only the important Mudras. For the instructions of all the Mudras, refer to my book "Hatha Yoga."

Instructions On Mudras And Bandhas

1. Maha Mudra, Maha Bandha and Maha Vedha form one group. They are something like three stages of one exercise. Similarly Mula Bandha, Uddiyana Bandha and Jalandhara Bandha form another group. Mula Bandha is practiced during Puraka, Kumbhaka, Rechaka, during meditation and Japa also. Uddiyana Bandha is practiced during Rechaka and Jalandhara Bandha during Kumbhaka.

2. As in the case of other Yogic Kriyas, Mudras and Bandhas also should be practiced when the stomach is empty. General instructions that are given for Asanas and Pranayamas should be followed for the practice of Mudras.

3. The benefits that are given may not be realized by the practice of Mudras alone. You will have to combine Pranayamas, Asanas, Japa and other Yogic Kriyas.

4. Khechari Mudra should be done under the direct guidance of a Khechari Guru. Cutting the lower tendon should be carefully done at regular intervals. Aspirants may not be successful in this Kriya if they begin after 25 years of age when the muscles and nerves have become stiff.

5. Khechari, Shakti Chalana, Vajroli and other advanced courses should not be practiced by all. The aspirants should ascertain from the Guru if they are fit for such advanced exercises and also they should see if they have all other requirements for the practice.

6. Uddiyana Bandha is also called Tadagi Mudra. Seet-Krama and Vyut-Krama described in the Neti Exercise are called Matangini Mudra. Do Mula Bandha. Release it. Again and again do like this. It is termed Aswini Mudra.

7. Those who have not undergone the preliminary portion of Khechari Mudra (making the tongue long) can simply keep the tongue turned upwards on the palate. This is Nabho Mudra or Manduki Mudra.

8. Real success in Mudras can be had only if there is intense concentration of mind. A detailed instruction on concentration will be given in the subsequent pages.

MISCELLANEOUS EXERCISES

Laya Yoga

Laya is the state of mind when one forgets all the objects of senses and gets absorbed in the object of meditation. Laya enables one to have perfect control over the five Tattvas, mind and Indriyas. The fluctuations of mind will stop. The mind, body and Prana will be entirely subdued.

For Laya Yoga, Sambhavi Mudra is an effective method, in which one intently concentrates on any one of the Shat Chakras. Trataka exercise plays a vital part in getting success in Laya. In due course of practice, the Yogin gets established in Samadhi. He becomes a Jivanmukta.

Anahata Sounds

Anahata sounds are the mystic sounds heard by the Yogin during his meditation. It is a sign of the purification of Nadis. Some students can clearly hear it through any one of the ears and some by both the ears. There are loud as well as subtle sounds. From the loud, one will have to contemplate on the subtle and from the subtle to the subtler. Beginners can hear the sound only when the ears are closed. Advanced students can concentrate on the Anahata sound even without closing the ears. Anahata sound is also termed Omkara Dhvani. They proceed from the Anahata center of the Sushumna Nadi.

Sit in your usual Asana. Close the ears with the thumbs. Hear and minutely observe the internal sound through the ears. The sound that you hear from within will make you deaf to all external sounds. Close the eyes also. In the beginning of your practice, you will hear many loud sounds. Later on they are heard in a mild way. The mind having at first concentrated itself on any one sound fixes firmly to that and is absorbed in it. The mind becoming insensible to the external impressions, becomes one with the sound as milk with water and then becomes rapidly absorbed in Chidakasa. Just as the bee drinking the honey alone does not care for the odor so also the Chitta, which is always absorbed in the inner sound, does not long for sensual objects, as it is bound by the sweet smell or Nada and has abandoned its flitting nature.

The sound proceeding from Pranava Nada, which is Brahman, is of the nature of effulgence. The mind gets absorbed in it. The mind exists so long as there is sound, but with its cessation, there is that state termed Turiya. It is the supreme state. It is the Unmani state. The mind gets absorbed along with Prana by constant concentration upon Nada. The body appears to be a log of wood and it does not feel heat or cold, joy or sorrow. Different kinds of sounds proceed from the heart (Anahata sounds).

Nada that is heard through the ears is of ten kinds. The first is the sound 'Chini' (like the pronunciation of the word); the second is 'Chini-chini'; the third is the sound of a bell; the fourth is that of a conch; the fifth is that of a lute; the sixth is the sound of cymbals; the seventh is the tune of a flute; the eighth is the voice of a drum (Bheri); the ninth is the sound of a double-drum (Mridanga); and the tenth is the sound of thunder.

You cannot expect the sound immediately after you close your ears. You should concentrate and keep your mind one-pointed. The particular sound that you hear today, you may not hear every day. But you will hear any one of the ten Anahata sounds.

The description given above is Laya through Nada, Anahata sound. In the same manner, Laya can be effected by concentration at the tip of the nose (Nasikagra Drishti), at the space between the two eyebrows (Bhrumadhya Drishti), meditation on the five Tattvas, on Soham Mantra, Aham Brahma Asmi, Tat Tvam Asi Mahavakyas and other methods also.

Bhakti Yoga — Classes Of Worship

At the lowest rung of the ladder of Bhakti Yoga comes the worship of elements and departed spirits. This is the lowest form of worship. Next comes the worship of Rishis, Devas and Pitris. The faith of each is shaped according to his own nature. The man consists of that which his faith is, he is even that. The third class includes those followers who worship Avataras like Sri Rama, Krishna, and Narasimha. The above four classes of Bhaktas have the Saguna form of worship. Next comes the class of Bhaktas who do Nirguna Upasana on Brahman devoid of attributes. This is the highest form of worship that is suitable for the intelligent people who have strong will and bold understanding. This is known as Ahamgraha Upasana or Jnana Yoga Sadhana.

Bhakti can be acquired and cultivated. Practice of the Nava Vidha Bhakti (nine methods of devotion) will infuse Bhakti. Constant Satsanga, Japa, Prayer, meditation, Svadhyaya, Bhajan, service to saints, Dana, Yatra, etc., will develop Bhakti. The following are the nine methods of developing Bhakti:

Sravana: —hearing of the Lilas of God
Smarana: —remembering God always

Kirtan: —singing His praise
Vandana: —Namaskaras to God
Archana: —offerings to God
Pada-Sevana: —attendance
Sakhya: —friendship
Dasya: —service
Atma-nivedana: —self-surrender to Guru or God

Sri Ramanuja recommends the following measures of developing Bhakti: —
Viveka: —discrimination
Vimoka: —freedom from all else and longing for God
Abhyasa: —continuous thinking of God
Kriya: —doing good to others
Kalyana: —wishing well to all
Satyam: —truthfulness
Arjavam: —integrity
Daya: —compassion
Ahimsa: —non-violence
Dana: —charity

Namdev, Ramdas, Tulsidas and others were a few blessed souls to whom God gave His Darshan. These Bhaktas were Yoga-Bhrashtas. They came into this world with a great asset of spiritual Samskaras. They worshipped God in several births with sincere devotion. They did not do much Sadhana in their final incarnation. This devotion was natural and spontaneous in them on account of the force of previous Samskaras of Bhakti. Ordinary people should adopt drastic, special measures and do special Sadhana for developing Bhakti rapidly. New grooves, new channels have to be cut in the old stony, devotionless heart to a maximum degree. Through constant prayer, Japa, Kirtan, service to Bhaktas, charity, Vrata, Tapas, Dhyana and

Samadhi a Bhakta should raise his consciousness to a high degree and acquire Para Bhakti, highest knowledge and Supreme peace. In the advanced stages of meditation, the meditator and the meditated, the worshipper and the worshipped, the Upasaka and the Upasya will become one. Dhyana will terminate in Samadhi. Constant and regular practice is necessary.

A Hatha Yogi reaches the highest stage by the practice of various Mudras, Bandhas, Asanas and other exercises; a Jnani by the practice of Sravana, Manana and Nididhyasana; a Karma Yogin by the selfless works (Nishkama Seva); a Bhakta by developing Bhakti and self-surrender, and a Raja Yogi by deep concentration and manipulation of the mind. The Goal is the same in all cases but the methods are different.

Concentration and meditation on the primordial energy, Shakti, is only a modification of Jnana Yogic Sadhana. Concentration and meditation on the different centers of energy belongs to Raja Yoga. Concentration at the different Chakras and Nadis and awakening the Shakti through physical methods belong to Hatha Yoga. Concentration and meditation on the Devata, presiding deity of the different inner Chakras, may be taken as an advanced course in Bhakti Yoga. For quick success, different methods of Sadhana should be combined.

The Bhakta when he meditates on the presiding deity or Devata imagines a particular form of God at each Chakra. In books of Mantra Shastra, elaborate descriptions of God and the Devatas are given for each Chakra. According to the temperament of the students they take the form of God in a different way. The experiences and feelings of the aspirants vary in all cases. Therefore I am not giving the descriptions of all the Devas and Devatas. When a man closes his eyes and meditates on the inner Chakras, he gets various visions and sees the different forms of God. That is the best to which he should cling. Then only real growth is possible. The general information that is given in the theoretical portion of this Kundalini Yoga will surely help a lot in concentration and meditation on the Chakras.

Mantras

Awakening Kundalini is effected by Mantra also. It is a portion of Bhakti Yoga. Some aspirants should repeat the Mantra given by their Guru even lakhs of times. During the time of Diksha of an Uttama Adhikari, the Guru utters a particular Mantra and Kundalini is awakened immediately. The consciousness of the student is raised to a very high degree. This depends upon the faith of the student in his Guru and in the Mantra. Mantras, when received from the Guru in person, are very powerful. Aspirants in Kundalini Yoga should take to this Mantra Sadhana only after getting a proper Mantra from a Guru. Therefore I am not touching this point in detail. Mantras when learnt through ordinary friends or through books cannot produce any benefit at all. Mantras are numerous and the Guru should select a particular Mantra by which the consciousness of a particular student can be awakened.

Eight Major Siddhis

An accomplished, Purnayogi in the path of Kundalini Yoga is in possession of eight major Siddhis, viz., Anima, Mahima, Laghima, Garima, Prapti, Prakamya, Vasitvam and Ishitvam.

1. *Anima*: The Yogi can become as minute as he pleases.

2. *Mahima*: This is the opposite of Anima. He can become as big as he likes. He can make his body assume a

very large size. He can fill up the whole universe. He can assume a Virat Svarupa.

3. *Laghima*: He can make his body as light as cotton or feather. Vayustambhanam is done through this Siddhi. In Jalastambhanam also the power is exercised to a very small degree. The body is rendered light by Plavini Pranayama. The Yogi produces a diminution of his specific gravity by swallowing large draughts of air. The Yogi travels in the sky with the help of this Siddhi. He can travel thousands of miles in a minute.

4. *Garima*: This is the opposite of Laghima. In this the Yogi acquires an increase of specific gravity. He can make the body as heavy as a mountain by swallowing draughts of air.

5. *Prapti*: The Yogi standing on the earth can touch the highest things. He can touch the sun or the moon or the sky. Through this Siddhi the Yogi attains his desired objects and supernatural powers. He acquires the power of predicting future events, the power of clairvoyance, clairaudience, telepathy, thought reading, etc. He can understand the languages of the beasts and birds. He can understand unknown languages also. He can cure all diseases.

6. *Prakamya*: He can dive into the water and can come out at any time he likes. The late Trilinga Swami of Benares used to live for six months underneath the Ganges. It is the process by which a Yogi makes himself invisible sometimes. By some writers it is defined to be the power of entering body of another (Parakaya Pravesh). Sri Sankara entered the body of Raja Amaruka of Benares. Tirumular in Southern India entered the body of a shepherd. Raja Vikramaditya also did this. It is also the power of keeping a youth-like appearance for any length of time. Raja Yayati had this power.

7. *Vashitvam*: This is the power of taming wild animals and bringing them under control. It is the power of mesmerizing persons by the exercise of will and of making them obedient to one's own wishes and orders. It is the restraint of passions and emotions. It is the power to bring men, women and the elements under subjection.

8. *Ishitvam*: It is the attainment of divine power. The Yogi becomes the Lord of the universe. The Yogi who has this power can restore life to the dead. Kabir, Tulsidas, Akalkot Swami and others had this power of bringing back life to the dead.

Minor Siddhis

The Yogi acquires the following minor Siddhis also:

1. Freedom from hunger and thirst.
2. Freedom from the effects of heat and cold.
3. Freedom from Raga-Dvesha.
4. Doora Darshan, clairvoyance or Dooradrishti.
5. Doora Sravan, clairaudience or Doora Sruti and Doora Pravachana.
6. Mano-Jaya, control of mind.
7. Kama Rupa: The Yogi can take any form he likes.
8. Parakaya Pravesha: He can enter into another body, can animate a dead body and enter into it by transferring his soul.
9. Iccha-Mrityu: Death at his will.
10. Devanam Saha Kreeda and Darshana: Playing with the gods after seeing them.
11. Yatha Sankalpa: Can get whatever he likes.
12. Trikala-Jnana: Knowledge of past, present and future.
13. Advandva: Beyond the pairs of opposites.
14. Vak-Siddhi: Whatever the Yogi predicts will come to pass by the practice of Satya, Prophecy.
15. The Yogi can turn base metal into gold.

16. Kaya-Vyuha: Taking as many bodies as the Yogi likes to exhaust all his Karmas in one life.

17. Darduri-Siddhi: The jumping power of a frog.

18. Patala-Siddhi: Yogi becomes Lord of desire, destroys sorrows and diseases.

19. He gets knowledge of his past life.

20. He gets knowledge of the cluster of stars and planets.

21. He gets the power of perceiving the Siddhas.

22. He gets mastery of the elements (Bhuta Jaya), mastery of Prana (Prana Jaya).

23. Kamachari: He can move to any place he likes.

24. He gets omnipotence and omniscience.

25. Vayu-Siddhi: The Yogi rises in the air and leaves the ground.

26. He can point out the place where a hidden treasure lies.

Power Of A Yogi

A Yogi forgets the body in order to concentrate the mind on the Lord. He conquers heat and cold by mastering breath-control and by controlling his nervous system.

A Yogi generates psychic heat in the body through the practice of Bhastrika Pranayama.

He can bear extremes of climates without discomfort.

He sits on the snow and melts it by the warmth generated in his body.

A Yogi covers his body with a sheet dipped in very cold water and dries it by the Yoga heat given off from his body. A few adepts have dried as many as thirty sheets in a single night.

A perfect Yogi cremates his body in the end by the Yogic heat generated by his power of Yoga.

Instructions On Siddhis

1. By the process of Hatha Yoga, the Yogi attains perfect physical body—*Rupalavanya Bala Vajrasam-hanana Kaya Sampat.* "The perfection of the body consists in beauty, grace, strength and adamantine hardness." The power to bear extreme cold and heat (Titiksha), the power to live without water and food and other powers come under the category of Kaya Sampat (perfection of body).

2. Since the body of the Hatha Yogi is perfect and firm, his mind also is firm and one-pointed. By the practices of Dharana and Dhyana, he reaches the highest rung in the Yogic ladder and attains Immortality through Yogic Samadhi. The Yogi, who has reached the highest stage, will have the 8 major and all the minor Siddhis.

3. Attainment of powers depends upon the amount of concentration at different Chakras and Tattvas and awakening of Kundalini. The practice of Mudras, Bandhas, Asanas and Pranayamas will also help a lot in acquiring Siddhis.

4. The Siddhis that are obtained by the practice of Mudras can be obtained by the practice of Bandhas, Asanas, Pranayamas and also by the concentration on different Chakras. That depends upon the temperament and capacity of the aspirants. One can obtain the desired goal by one exercise and others by different methods. Therefore if one is not able to get success by a particular exercise, he will have to have recourse to other exercises.

5. Many of the 8 major Siddhis are not possible at all at the present age (Kali Yuga), when the body and mind of the vast majority are not fit enough. Even today there are several Siddhas who have the power to perform some of the Siddhis. When people approach them to do this and that, they hide themselves or generally say: —"I do not know." They are not much particular about these Siddhis.

Their aim is to ignore these as unreal and aspire to reach the highest. They are the only real Yogins. Many are able to use some powers and they do not know how they are able to do them.

6. One can read the thoughts of others. A man in London hears the spiritual message of sages in India. You have seen several persons removing the poison of cobras by chanting some Mantras or by mere touch. By giving some sort of leaves, incurable diseases are cured. There are men who will very accurately tell your past, present and future. Some are able to see astral entities. Stopping the functions of the heart and changing the mind of others and other powers are due to Yogic practices.

7. Nowadays you cannot find a man who has developed all the powers. When one gets certain powers, he stops there by the influence of Maya and false Tushti (satisfaction) and uses the powers for his livelihood or for fame. Therefore he is not able to proceed further and attain perfection. It is not the mistake of the Yogic Kriyas. You should not lose faith. Faith, attention, sincerity and earnestness will lead you to success.

Dharana (Concentration)

1. Fix the mind on some object either within the body or outside. Keep it there steady for some time. This is Dharana. You will have to practice this daily. Laya-Yoga has its basis on Dharana.

2. Purify the mind first through the practice of Yama, Niyama and then take to the practice of Dharana. Concentration without purity is of no use. There are some occultists who have concentration. But they have no good character. That is the reason why they do not make any progress in the spiritual line.

3. He who has a steady Asana and has purified the Yoga Nadis will be able to concentrate easily. Concentration will be intense if you remove all distractions. A true Brahmachari, who has preserved his Veerya, will have wonderful concentration.

4. Some foolish, impatient students take to Dharana at once without undergoing the preliminary ethical training. This is a serious blunder. Ethical perfection is of paramount importance.

5. You can concentrate internally on any one of the seven Chakras and externally on any Devata, Hari, Krishna or Devi.

6. Attention plays a prominent part in concentration. He who has developed his power of attention will have good concentration. A man, who is filled with passion and all sorts of fantastic desires, can hardly concentrate on any object even for a second. His mind will be jumping like a monkey.

7. He who has gained Pratyahara (withdrawing the senses from the objects) will have a good concentration. You will have to march in the spiritual path step-by-step, stage-by-stage. Lay the foundation of Yama, Niyama, Asana, Pranayama and Pratyahara to start with. The super-structure of Dharana and Dhyana will be successful only then.

8. You should be able to visualize very clearly the object of concentration even in its absence. You must call up the mental picture at a moment's notice. If you have good practice in concentration, you can do this without much difficulty.

9. In the beginning stage of practice, you can concentrate on the tick-tick sound of a watch or on the flame of the candle or on any other object that is pleasing to the mind. This is concrete concentration. There can be

no concentration without something upon which the mind may rest. The mind can be fixed on a pleasant object. It is very difficult in the beginning to fix the mind on any object which it dislikes.

10. If you want to increase your power of concentration you will have to reduce your worldly activities. You will have to observe Mouna everyday for two hours or even more.

11. Practice concentration till the mind is well established on the object of concentration. When the mind runs away from the object, bring it back again.

12. When concentration is deep and intense, all other senses cannot operate. He who practices concentration for one hour daily has tremendous psychic powers. He will have a strong will power.

13. Vedantins try to fix the mind on Atman. This is their Dharana. Hatha Yogins and Raja Yogins concentrate their mind on the six Chakras. Bhaktas concentrate on their Ishta Devata. Other objects of meditation are described under Trataka and Laya Yoga. Concentration is necessary for all the aspirants.

14. Those who practice concentration evolve quickly. They can do any work with greater efficiency in no time. What others can do in six hours can be done easily in half an hour by one who has a concentrated mind. Concentration purifies and calms the surging emotions, strengthens the current of thought and clarifies the ideas. Concentration keeps a man in his material progress also. He will turn out very good work in his office or business-house. What was cloudy and hazy before becomes clearer and definite; What was very difficult before becomes easy now; and what was complex, bewildering and confusing before, comes easily within the mental grasp. You can achieve anything by concentration. Nothing is impossible for one who regularly

practices concentration. Clairvoyance, clairaudience, mesmerism, hypnotism, thought reading, music, mathematics and other sciences depend upon concentration.

15. Retire into a quiet room. Close your eyes. See what happens when you think of an apple. You may think of its color, shape, size, different parts such as skin, pulp, seeds, etc. You may think of the places, Australia or Kashmir, wherefrom it is imported. You may think of its acidic or sweet taste and its effects on the digestive system and blood. Through the law of association, ideas of some other fruits also may try to enter. The mind may begin to entertain some other extraneous ideas. It may begin to wander. It may think of meeting a friend at the Railway Station at 4 p.m. It may think of purchasing a towel or a tin of tea or biscuits. You should try to have a definite line of thought. There should not be any break in the line of thinking. You must not entertain any other thought which is not connected with the subject on hand. The mind will try its level best to run in its old grooves. You will have to struggle hard in the beginning. The attempt is somewhat like going up a steep hill. You will rejoice and feel immense happiness when you get success in concentration.

16. Just as laws of gravitation, cohesion, etc., operate in the physical plane, so also definite laws of thought such as laws of association, relativity, contiguity, etc., operate in the mental plane or thought-world. Those who practice concentration should thoroughly understand these laws. When the mind thinks of an object, it may think of its qualities and its parts also. When it thinks of a cause it may think of its effect also.

17. If you read with concentration Bhagavad Gita or the Vicar of Wakefield several times, you can get new ideas each time. Through concentration you will get insight.

Subtle esoteric meanings will flash out in the field of mental consciousness. You will understand the inner depth of philosophical significance.

18. When you concentrate on an object do not wrestle with the mind. Avoid tension anywhere in the body. Think gently of the object in a continuous manner. It is very difficult to practice concentration when one is very hungry and when one is suffering from an acute disease.

19. If emotions disturb you during concentration, do not mind them. They will pass away soon. If you try to drive them away you will have to tax your will-force. Have an indifferent attitude. To drive the emotions away, the Vedantin uses the formula: "I am a Sakshi of the mental modifications. I don't care. Get out". The Bhakta simply prays, and help comes from God.

20. Train the mind in concentrating on various objects, gross and subtle, of various sizes. In course of time a strong habit will be formed. The moment you sit for concentration, the mood will come at once, quite easily.

21. When you read a book you must read with concentration. There is no use of skipping over the pages in a hurried manner. Read one page. Close the book. Concentrate on what you have read. Find out parallel lines in Gita, Upanishads, etc.

22. For a neophyte the practice of concentration is disgusting and tiring in the beginning. He has to cut new grooves in the mind and brain. After some time, say two or three months, he gets great interest. He enjoys a new kind of happiness. Concentration is the only way to get rid of the miseries and tribulations. Your only duty is to achieve concentration and through concentration to attain the final beatitude, Self-realization. Charity and Rajasuya Yajna are nothing when compared with concentration.

23. When desires arise in the mind, do not try to fulfill them. Reject them as soon as they arise. Thus by gradual practice the desires can be reduced. The modifications of the mind will also diminish a lot.

24. You must get rid of all sorts of mental weakness, superstitions, false and wrong Samskaras. Then only you will be able to concentrate your mind.

Chapter Six

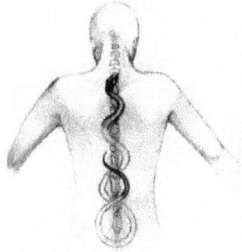

YOGA ADDENDA

1. Sadasiva Brahman

Sri Sadasiva Brahman, a reputed Yogi, lived in Nerur, near Karur, in Trichinopolly district, some one hundred and twenty years ago. He was the author of 'Atma Vilas', 'Brahma Sutras' and various other works. Once he was in Samadhi. The floods in the Cauveri River covered him up with mud. For some months his body remained buried underneath the earth. The agriculturists tilled the land and injured the head of the Yogi. Some blood oozed out. They were quite astonished. They dug out the earth. Sadasiva Brahman got up from his Samadhi and walked away. Once some rude people came with sticks to beat him. They raised their hands, but they were not able to move them. They remained like statues. At some other time he entered the Zenana of a Nawab quite naked while he was roaming about as an Avadhuta. The Nawab got enraged and cut off his hand with a big knife. Sadasiva Brahman went away with a laugh. The Nawab thought that the man should be a great Sage. He took the maimed hand and followed the Sage. On the third day the Nawab said: "O my Lord! I cut off your hand due to my foolishness. Kindly forgive me."

Sadasiva simply touched the cut portion with the other hand. There was a new hand. Sadasiva forgave the Nawab and blessed him.

2. Jnanadev

Sri Jnanadev is also known as Jnaneswar. He was the greatest Yogin the world has ever produced. He was born in Alandi, 7 miles from Poona. His Samadhi is there even now. If anybody reads the Gita written by him by the side of the Samadhi all the doubts are cleared. He is regarded as an Avatara of Lord Krishna. When he was a boy he simply touched a buffalo. It repeated the Vedas. He had full control over the elements. When there was no vessel to prepare food, his sister prepared bread on his back. He entered Samadhi while alive at the age of 22. He drew up all the Prana to the Brahmarandhra and gave up the physical body. When he was a boy of 14 years, he began to write commentary on Gita. His commentary on Gita is considered one of the best. In a big assembly of Sanskrit Pandits in Benares, he was selected President.

3. Trilinga Swami

Sri Trilinga Swami of Benares, born in Andhra Desa, lived some fifty years ago. He lived for 280 years. He made his Tapas in Manasarovar (Tibet). Once Ramakrishna Paramahamsa also saw him at Benares. He brought some money to Benares when he first came in for Tapas. He opened a milk-shop and distributed milk free to poor persons, Sadhus and Sannyasins. He used to live underneath the Ganga water even for six months continuously. He used to sleep in Kashi Visvanath's Temple keeping his feet over the Sivalinga. Once he caught hold of the sword of the Governor and threw it into the Ganges. When the Governor demanded it back, he dived into the water and brought back two swords and the Governor was unable to find out his own sword. Some mischief-makers poured some limewater in his mouth. He at once pumped it out through the anus by Sang Pachar Kriya.

4. Gorakhnath

Sri Gorakhnath was a great Yogi like Sri Jnanadev of Alandi. In Chandragiri village on the banks of the Godavari, there was a Brahmin named Suraj. His wife's name was Sarasvati. They had no children. Yogi Matsyendranath went for Bhiksha in the house of Suraj. Sarasvati entertained the Yogi with good food, with Sraddha. She wept before him for not having a child. Yogi Matsyendranath gave her a pinch of holy ash with blessings for a child. Some time later, she had a son. Matsyendranath came back to Sarasvati and took the boy with him when he was twelve years of age. He sent the boy to Badrinarayan for doing Tapas. Apsaras and other Devatas came to molest him. He stood firm and tided over all temptations. He got tremendous Siddhis. Matsyendranath also imparted all his powers and Vidyas to the boy, his disciple, Gorakhnath.

Sri Gorakhnath in his 12th year went to Badrinarayan and performed Tapas for 12 long years, living on air alone. Gorakhnath had tremendous Yogic powers. When his Guru Matsyendranath entered the dead body of a Raja (Parakaya Pravesh) to obey the orders of Sri Hanuman to produce an offspring for a certain Rani, Gorakhnath assumed the form of a lady through his Yogic powers and entered the inner apartments of the palace (Kamarupa Siddhi). At some other instance he made a toy child out of clay and gave this as a playmate for the children of a certain village. He converted a portion of a mountain into gold and reconverted it to its former condition. He passed urine on a rock. It became gold. Once in a Kumbhamela on the banks of the Godavari, he gave food to all by spreading only leaves but offered different rich meals to the liking of everyone. In the same Mela he slowly reduced himself in bulk and assumed the form of a mosquito (Anima Siddhi). Through his own Yogic power he burnt himself to ashes and again assumed his original form. He did Akasagamanam (walking in the sky). In this way he performed many Siddhis. Raja Bhartrihari was his disciple.

5. Swami Krishna Ashram

Swami Krishna Ashram is a living saint at Daroli village, 14 miles below Gangotri, the origin of the Ganges. He has been living there for the last eight years in an absolutely nude state, in an icy region, where an ordinary man may require a woolen sweater, a Gothma and half a dozen blankets. He was a Siva Bhakta. He threw away all his Puja-vessels, went to Varanasi, took Sannyasa and lived there for a year. Then he went to Hardwar, threw off the Danda and became an Avadhuta. He was in Uttarkashi also. When sharp, big flies were biting his body, when blood was emerging profusely, he would never disturb the flies. Such was his power of endurance. Once in the Kshetra an arrogant servant insulted him for not bringing any vessel for Dhal and poured very hot Dhal on his hands. Swami Krishna Ashram drank the Dhal though his lips and hands were scalded. There is another Swami by name Bhuma Ashram, living at Daroli in a nude state. He is a friend of Krishna Ashram.

Titiksha, the power of endurance, is an essential attribute of all Sadhakas. This is one of the six fold virtues of Sadhana Chatushtaya. Read Slokas 14 and l5 of the Gita, Chapter II. You will understand the importance of this virtue, Titiksha.

6. Yogi Bhusunda

Yogi Bhusunda is one of the Chiranjivis amongst the Yogins. He was the master in the science of Pranayama. It is said that a big nest, like a mountain, was built by him on the southern branch of the Kalpa Vriksha, situated at the northern summit of the Mahameru. Bhusunda lived in this nest. He was a Trikala Jnani. He could sit in Samadhi for any length of time. He was desireless. He had obtained supreme Santi and Jnana. He was there enjoying the bliss of his own Self and he is still there being a Chiranjivi. He had the full knowledge of the five Dharanas. He had rendered himself proof against the five elements by practicing the five methods of concentration. It is said that when all the twelve Adityas scorch the world with their burning rays, he would, through his Apas Dharana, reach up the Akasa. When fierce gales arise splintering up the rocks to pieces, he would be in the Akasa through Agni Dharana. When the world together with the Mahameru would be under water, he would float on them through Vayu Dharana.

7. Tirumula Nayanar

Tirumula Nayanar was a great Yogi in Kailas. He had all the 8 major Siddhis through the grace of Nandi, the Vahana of Lord Siva. He was a friend of Agastya Muni. He came from Kailas and stayed in Varanasi. Then he went to Chidambaram and Tiruvavaduturai and other places near Madras. He worshipped Lord Siva in the temple at Tiruvavaduturai and stayed there for some time. Once he went to a garden on the banks of the river Cauveri. There he saw the dead body of a caretaker of a herd of cows. He noticed that all the cows surrounded the dead body of the cowherd and were crying bitterly. This touched the heart of Tirumular. He pitied the cows very much. He left his body in a certain place and entered the dead body of the cowherd. He looked after the cows throughout the day and sent them back to their respective houses. The wife of the cowherd, who was not aware of the death of her husband, invited Tirumular who was wearing the physical body of her husband. Tirumular refused. He wanted to enter his own body. When he searched for his body, it was not found in the original place. Then he thought it was all the grace of Lord Siva. Then with the body of the cowherd, he went to Avaduturai and sat underneath an Asvattha tree on the western side of the temple and wrote a valuable book called "Tirumantram" in Tamil. It is a book of 3000 verses which contain the essence of the Vedas.

8. Mansoor

Mansoor was a Sufist Brahma-Jnani. He lived in Persia, some four hundred years ago. He was repeating always "Anal-haq! Anal-haq!" This corresponds to "Soham" or "Aham Brahma Asmi" of the Vedantins. People reported to the Badshah that Mansoor was an atheist (Kafir) and that he was always uttering "Anal-haq." The Badshah was quite enraged. He ordered that Mansoor must be cut into pieces. His orders were obeyed. Even then the pieces of flesh were uttering "Anal-haq." He felt no pain as he was a full-blown Samadhi Jnani and as he had full identification with Brahman. He above body-consciousness. Then they put the pieces of flesh and bones in the fire and reduced them into ashes. Even then the ashes uttered "Anal-haq." During his lifetime he performed many miracles. Even Jnanis can do miracles if they desire and if they find it necessary for the occasion. Sadasiva Brahman and other Jnanis did wonders. Remember the lives of great men daily. You will advance in the spiritual path.

9. Milarepa

Milarepa was one who had been profoundly impressed from his youth by the transient and impermanent nature of all conditions of worldly existence and by the sufferings and wretchedness in which he saw all beings immersed. To him existence seemed like a huge furnace where all living creatures were roasting. With such piercing sorrow did this fill his heart that he was unable to feel even any of the celestial felicity enjoyed by Brahma and Indra in their heavens, much less of the earthly joys and delights afforded by a life of worldly greatness.

On the other hand, he was so captivated by the vision of immaculate purity, by the chaste beauty in the description of the state of perfect freedom and omniscience associated with the attainment of Nirvana, that he cared not even though he might lose his very life in the search on which he had set out, endowed as he was with full faith, keen intellect and a heart overflowing with all-pervading love and sympathy to all.

Having obtained transcendental knowledge in the control of the ethereal and spiritual nature of the mind, he was enabled to furnish demonstration thereof by flying through the sky, by walking, resting and sleeping on the air. Likewise he was able to produce flames of fire and springs of water from his body and to transform his body at will into any object desired, thereby convincing unbelievers and turning them towards religious pursuits.

He was perfect in the practice of the four stages of meditation and thus he was able to project his subtle body so as to be present as the presiding Yogi in twenty-four holy places where gods and angels assemble, like clouds for spiritual communion.

He was able to dominate gods and elementals and make them carry out his commands instantaneously, in the fulfillment of all duties. He was a perfect adept in supernatural powers. He was able to transverse and visit all the innumerable sacred paradises and heavens of the Buddhas, where by virtue of his all-absorbing acts of unsurpassed devotion the Buddhas and Bodhisattvas presiding therein favored him with discourses on Dharma and listened to his in return, so that he sanctified the heaven-worlds by his visits and sojourns there.

10. Napoleon Bonaparte

Napoleon Bonaparte was a man of great concentration. His success was all due to the power of concentration. He suffered from various diseases as epileptic fits, Brady cardia, etc. But for these maladies, he would have proved still more powerful. He could sleep at any time he liked. He would snore the very moment he retired to bed. He would get up at the very second of the appointed time. This is a kind of Siddhi. He had no Vikshepa or shilly-shallying. He had the highly developed Ekagrata of a Yogi. He could draw, as it were, any single thought from the brain pigeonhole, dwell on it as long as he liked and could shove it back when finished. He would sleep very soundly at night amidst busy war, would never worry a bit at night. This was all due to his power of concentration. Concentration can do anything. Without concentration of mind nothing can be achieved.

Messrs. Gladstone and Balfour had a great deal of concentration of mind. The very moment they retired to bed, they would get sleep. Mark the word "very moment". They would never toss about for 15 or 20 minutes in the bed as in the case of the worldly persons. Think how difficult it is to enter into deep sleep the very moment you lie down. They had perfect control over sleep. They could also get up from bed at any time they wished without any alarm timepiece. Sleeping and getting up at the appointed second is only an example to show the power of concentration to a certain degree. There are people who, after a day's hard work, can sleep the very moment they go to bed; but they cannot get up at the appointed time. This is only an example on a very ordinary thing. People of concentration can work wonders and miracles.

11. Teachings Of Kabir

Once Kabir tied a stout pig to the front post in the verandah of his house. An orthodox Brahmin Pundit came to Kabir's house for discussing a philosophical problem. He saw the pig in front of the house. He was much upset, irritated and annoyed. He asked Kabir: —"Dear Sir, how is it you have tied a nasty animal that eats the excreta of human beings, very close to your house. You have no Achara. You are a dirty man. You do not know the Shastras. You are ignorant". Kabir replied: —"O Shastriji, you are more dirty than myself. I have tied the pig to the front post outside my house, whereas you have tied the pig to the mind". The Brahmin was very much vexed and went away without telling a word. *Man changa katorie me ganga*: "If the mind is pure, you will find the Ganges in the cup". Purification of mind is of paramount importance. Without this nothing can be achieved in the spiritual path.

12. A Sham Latin Scholar

A certain man went to a Latin teacher to learn Latin. He stayed with the teacher for a week. He noticed that most of the words ended in 'o'. He thought that he must add the letter 'o' to the end of each word. He knew English well. He told the teacher that he knew Latin and with the permission of the teacher, he went back to his native place. He reached his house and tapped the door uttering these words: —"O, dear-o, wife-o, open-o, door-o". He thought this was all Latin.

There are very many scholars in Yoga and Vedanta also similar to the learned Latin scholar, above narrated. They stay for a few days in Ram Ashram Library or with some Sadhus, learn the names Kundalini, Mula Chakra, Nadi, Pranayama, Maya, or Pratibimbavada and move from place to place. Yoga and Vedanta are philosophies that are to be studied under a Guru with great interest for a period of 12 years. Then only one can master the subjects. Yoga and Vedanta should not be used as a means for livelihood. After learning a few words in Yoga and Vedanta, one should not go about and mix with the worldly people. Attaining perfection in Yoga requires a long practical experience under a perfect guide.

13. Story Of An Aspirant

An aspirant went to a Mahant of Gorakhnath Panth. Gorakhnath-followers are those who wear either big black celluloid or glass earrings. The Mahant bored the aspirant's ears, inserted big earrings and gave him a beautiful name also, Yogi Ishvarananda. He remained in the Ashram for three months. He did not get any spiritual progress. He thought to himself: —"This is not the proper path. Let me try another path." He left the Ashram immediately, wandered through thick jungles, came across a Fakir and implored for initiation. The Fakir circumcised, gave him a Mantra and asked him to have a long beard. This also did not satisfy him. Now look at the pitiable condition of this poor aspirant. The ulcers in the ears had not healed up properly. He had considerable pain through septic inflammation. There was profuse discharge of pus. He had already a disturbed state of mind and this state of affairs augmented his mental worries. He seriously reflected that this was not the way of seeking the Guru. He made a strong determination that he must not roam about, must stick firmly to one solitary place and must perform their Tapas with constant prayers to God. He selected a place and performed Tapas with all sincerity. This purified him and made him fit for higher steps. After a period of two years, a Guru appeared before him, initiated him into deep mysteries of Yoga. Present-day aspirants also are running like this from place to place in search of a Guru. It is of no use. They should purify themselves for a Yogic life. By chance, even if they come in contact with an Avatara, they will not be benefited much if they have not a strong foundation for a Yogic life.

14. Other Yogins

The yogi by means of various practices establishes a conscious control over the organs and functions of the body. He moulds his body like steel. One Swami in London had a demonstration of stopping his heart before the King. Many able physicians were present on the occasion and examined him. Desabandhu in 1926 stopped the radial and temporal pulses on both sides at will and stopped the beatings of the heart also for a short time. He showed a demonstration in the Bombay Medical Union. In Maharajah Ranjit Singh's Court in Lahore, Hatha Yogi Hari Das who buried himself underneath the ground for forty days after tightly closing his nose, mouth, ears and eyes with wax came back alive. The Mohammedan Yogi, Gunangudi Mastan, was buried in Madras. Some Yogins fly in the air. This is due to Khechari Mudra.

Yogi Pratap was in the posture of doing Viparitakarani Mudra. He asked the onlookers to cover his head with clay on all sides. He remained in that position for full 2 hours. Paul Deussen, the German traveler, personally witnessed this in Varanasi. Sri Swami Vishuddhananda of Varanasi once gave life to a dead sparrow. Nothing is impossible for a real Yogi.

Mystic Experience—Visions Of Lights

Various kinds of lights manifest during meditation owing to deep concentration. In the beginning a bright, white light, the size of a pin's point will appear in the forehead at the space between the two eyebrows which corresponds tentatively to the Ajna Chakra. You will notice, when the eyes are closed, different colored lights, white, yellow, red, smoky, blue, green, mixed lights, flashes like lightning, fire, moon, sun, stars and sparks. These are Tanmatric lights. Each Tanmatra has its own specific color. Yellow and white lights are very commonly seen. In the beginning small balls of white or red light float about before the mind's eye. When you first observe this be assured that the mind is becoming steadier and that you are progressing in concentration. After some months, the size of the light will increase and you will see a full blaze of white light, bigger than the sun. In the beginning these lights are not steady. They come and disappear immediately. When you have steady and systematic practice of meditation for 2 or 3 hours, these lights appear more frequently and remain steady for a long time. The vision of lights is a great encouragement in Sadhana. It impels you to stick to Sadhana steadily. It gives you strong faith in superphysical matter. The appearance of the lights denotes that you are transcending the physical consciousness. You are in a semiconscious state when the light appears. You are between the two places. You must not shake the body when these lights manifest. You must be perfectly steady in your Asana and breathe slowly.

At times you will see some lustrous forms of Devatas or some other physical forms. You will see your Ishta Devata or your Guru. Siddhas, Rishis and others give their Darshan to encourage you. You can see beautiful gardens, palatial buildings, rivers, mountains, golden temples, and sceneries so lovely and picturesque as cannot be adequately described.

During intense concentration, many are able to feel certain peculiar sensation as if some electric current passes from the Muladhara-Chakra. They immediately disturb their body and come down to the physical consciousness out of fear. They need have no fear at all. They should keep steady and wait for further experiences.

The experiences vary in different individuals. The experience of one man may not be the same as that of another man. Many erroneously believe that they have realized the Self when they get these experiences, stop their Sadhana and try to move with the public to preach and to do Loka-Sangraha. This is a serious blunder. This is not realization at all. These are all simple encouragements from your Ishta Devata to convince you of a higher spiritual life and push you in your systematic and incessant practice with zeal and enthusiasm. You will have to ignore these things and drive them away just as you did with worldly objects. You must not care a bit when you get these visions. You must have your Lakshya on the goal. The visions may appear in some persons within a few days, while in others within six or nine months. It depends upon the state of the mind and degree of concentration. Some persons may not have such experiences, but they will be progressing in the spiritual path.

Sometimes you will get very powerful, dazzling lights, bigger than the sun. They are white. In the beginning, they come and disappear quickly. Later on they become steady even for 10 or 15 minutes according to the degree of concentration. Lights will appear before the eyes or at any one of the Chakras. The light is so powerful and dazzling sometimes that you have to withdraw yourself from looking and break your meditation. Some people are afraid and they do not know what to do and how to proceed further. By constant practice, the mind engaged in concentration will vanish. The beings and objects with whom you are in touch during the early period of Sadhana belong to the astral world. The lustrous forms are higher Devatas of mental and higher planes, who come down to give Darshan and to encourage the Sadhakas. Various Shaktis manifest in lustrous forms. Adore them. Do mental Puja as soon as they appear before you.

Do not waste your time in looking at these visions. This is only a curiosity. These are all encouragements to convince you of the existence of superphysical, metaphysical realities. Visions are either subjective or objective, your own mental creations or of realities on finer planes of matter. Universe consists of planes of matter of various degrees of density. Rhythmical vibrations of Tanmatras in various degrees give rise to the formation of various planes. Visions may be of these things or beings. Or in many cases they may be purely imaginary. They may be the crystallization of your own intense thinking. You must discriminate well.

Elementals

Sometimes these elementals appear during meditation. They are strange figures, some with long teeth, big faces, some with three heads, some with faces on the belly, some without flesh and skin, etc. They are inhabitants of Bhuvar Loka. They are Bhutas. They are supposed to be the attendants of Lord Siva. They have terrifying forms.

They do not cause any harm at all. They simply appear on the stage. They come to test your strength and courage. They can do nothing. They cannot stand before a pure, ethical aspirant. Repetition of Om or your Guru Mantra will throw them at a distance. Whenever young people look at a dead body or when they see a body hanging or when they see a cruel murder, they always brood over this instance. Even during meditation, the same thought will come and take peculiar form. Again and again they will see the same form before their eyes. They should not fear at all. It is only their mental creation. A coward is absolutely unfit for the spiritual line. Destroy fear. Develop courage. Be bold.

Life In The Astral Plane

During the course of practice, one day you will feel that you have separated yourself from the body. You will have immense joy mixed with fear; joy in the possession of a new light, astral body; and fear owing to the entry in a foreign, unknown plane. At the very outset, the new consciousness is very rudimentary in the new plane. You will only feel that you have a light, airy body and will perceive a rotating, vibrating, limited astral atmosphere with illumination of golden lights, objects and beings. You may feel that you are floating in the air.

You will never fall; but the new experience of subtlety generates novel feelings and sensations in the beginning. How you leave the body and remain, is unknown. You are unaware of how you have completely separated yourself from the body. The new joy is inexpressible. Your will have to actually feel and experience it yourself. When you come back to body-consciousness, there is an intense craving to regain the new consciousness and to remain in that state always. By chance, by repeated attempts, you are able to go beyond the body-consciousness once in a month or so in the course of Sadhana. If you plod on with patience, through Yogic practices, you will be able to leave the body at will and stay for a long time.

You can by mere willing travel in any place you like with the astral body and there materialize by drawing the necessary materials either from Ahamkara or the universal storehouse. The process is very simple to occultists and Yogis who know the rationale, the detailed technique of the various operations. Those who can function with the astral body can very easily perform thought reading, thought-transference, psychic healing, distant healing, etc. Concentrated mental rays can penetrate opaque walls and travel miles and miles.

Hints On Yoga

Brahmacharya is very essential Even in dreams you must be free from lustful thoughts. It requires long practice and careful watch over the mind and Indriyas. Foolish people hastily jump up to the higher courses in Yoga in vain without having this important item which is very useful for spiritual Sadhana.

Wet dreams generally occur in the last quarter of the night. Those who are in the habit of getting up from bed between 3 and 4 a.m. (Brahmamuhurta) and doing Japa, Pranayama and Dhyana, can never fall a victim to nocturnal pollutions.

That man in whom the sex-idea is deep-rooted can never dream of understanding Yoga and Vedanta even in one hundred births.

Keep the mind fully occupied. This is the best panacea or sovereign remedy for keeping up Brahmacharya. Do Japa, meditation, reading of religious books, walking, Kirtan, prayer, Satsanga, service, religious discourse, writing, etc.

Always wear a Kaupeen or Langotee. This is scientific and spiritual too. If you are a married man, sleep in a separate room from your wife. Change your habit immediately.

Be careful in the selection of your companions. Give up drama, talkies, reading novels and other love-stories. Do not use soaps and flowers. Observe Mowna. Do not mix with anyone. Read good inspiring religious books. When desires arise in the mind do not fulfill them. Crush them immediately. Avoid the company of women. No joking and laughing. These are all outward manifestations of lust only. When you walk in the street do not look hither and thither like a monkey. Do not look at a woman—even the photo or picture of a lady. Do not talk about women.

When you advance in the spiritual practice it will be very difficult for you to do both meditation and daily office and household work at the same time, because the mind will undergo a double strain. It finds it very difficult to adjust to different uncongenial activities. Therefore, the advanced Grihastha-students will have to stop all worldly activities. When they advance in meditation, if they desire to advance further, they should take to seclusion and must disconnect themselves from the worldly activities entirely. Work is a hindrance in meditation for advanced Yogic students.

Live alone. Observe Mowna and record in your diary the benefits you derive. Do not make gestures and signs *hu, hu, hu*. This *hu, hu, hu* is tantamount to talking. There is more wastage of energy in this *hu, hu, hu* business. Utilize this conserved energy in Japa and meditation.

Sadhakas who take up to Nivritti Marga generally become lazy after some time, as they do not know how to utilize the mental energy, as they do not keep up any daily routine and as they do not follow the instructions of their Guru. They get Vairagya of course, but they have no experience in the spiritual line. They do not make any spiritual progress in the end.

Those who want to take up to seclusion and Nivritti Marga should observe Mowna and discipline the Indriyas, mind and body while living in the world. They should train themselves to hard, laborious life, coarse food, walking without shoes and umbrella. Then only they can bear the rigorous life of an ascetic. They should entirely give up timidity.

If circumstances prevent you from observing Mowna, strictly avoid long talk, big talk, tall talk and all sorts of vain discussions and withdraw yourself from society as much as possible. Too much of talk is simply wastage of energy. If this energy is conserved by Mowna, it will be transmuted into Ojas Shakti which will help you in your Sadhana.

Sadhaka should always remain alone. This is an important factor in spiritual progress. Mixing with householders is highly dangerous. Solitude for Sadhana is a great desideratum. All energies must be carefully preserved. After a short stay in solitude, aspirants should not enter the world. What they have gained in five years in seclusion through hard Tapas will be irrecoverably lost in a month by mixing with worldly people. Several persons have complained to me that they have lost the power of concentration.

After attaining perfection in Yoga, one can enter world if he is not affected even a bit by unfavorable, hostile currents of the world. There is no harm if you mix with congenial company which is also devoted to Yoga Abhyasa. You can discuss various philosophical points. You can be in the company of higher spiritual personages who enter into Samadhi. Many persons enter the world before perfection in Yoga to demonstrate their minor powers in the name of Loka Sangraha and for fame. They have been reduced to a level worse than a worldly man.

Everything must be done gradually. It is very difficult for a man who was in the world to be in entire seclusion. It will be very painful and troublesome for a beginner. He should slowly train himself by observing Mowna often.

The place wherein you can get concentration of mind is suitable for your Yogic practices. This is a general rule. There will be no use if you run from place to place.

When you do Karma Yoga you must be free from egoism. You must not expect any reward or appreciation for the work that you do (Nishkama). You must have a balanced mind in success and failure. The moment the Chitta-Shuddhi is attained, you must stop doing Nishkama Karma and take to pure meditation in seclusion.

Most of the difficulties arise in your daily life if you do not have a proper control over your mind. For instance, if a man does evil to you, instantly you want to revenge, to extract tooth for tooth, tit for tat policy, to return anger for anger. Every reaction of evil shows that the mind is not under control. By anger one loses his energy. Balanced state of mind is not possible. From anger all other impurities emanate. Anger controlled properly, becomes transmuted into an energy so powerful as to move the whole world.

A slight overloading in the stomach will upset meditation. The mind has direct connection with gastric nerves of the stomach. You will get drowsiness also. You must train yourself to 'Mitahara'.

When you have diet restriction, in the beginning you will imagine that you are getting leaner and weaker. To add to this your friends and relatives will frighten you. Do not hear them. In a few days you will be quite all right.

In case of indigestion and constipation, take a long brisk walk in the morning. As soon as you get up from bed drink large quantity of water. Do Paschimottana, Mayura, Trikona Asanas, Nauli and Uddiyana. Do physical exercises also. In case of chronic constipation try a change in diet. If you take rice, then take wheat, and see. If you are in the same state, try fruits and milk diet. Then you will be quite all right. Change of diet is a sure remedy.

If you have the evil habit of drinking wine, toddy, coffee, etc., and if you want to stop it, go to the meditation room and promise before the deity that you will stop the bad habit from that moment. Proclaim this determination to your friends. If your mind goes to the same habit, you will naturally be ashamed to continue the habit. Several times you will fail. Still struggle hard. Take to Satsanga. Study religious books. You can destroy all impure habits. If you find it very difficult to give up, the last remedy you will have to take is in running away from the present society and you must flee to a place where you cannot at all get all these. Out of compulsion you can leave the bad habit.

If you want to stop taking mutton, fish etc., just see with your own eyes the pitiable, struggling condition at the time of killing the sheep or fish. Now mercy and sympathy will arise in your heart. Then you will determine to give up flesh eating so that the poor innocent lives may be spared. If you fail in this attempt, just change your environments and live in a Brahmin hotel where you cannot get mutton and fish and move with that society where there is only vegetable diet. Always think of the evils of flesh eating and the benefits of vegetable diet. If this also cannot give you sufficient strength to stop this habit, go to the slaughterhouse and butcher's shop and personally see the disgusting rotten muscles, kidneys and other nasty parts of the animal and the bad smell. This will induce Vairagya in you and a strong disgust and hatred for mutton eating.

A Mantra is a mass of Tejas or radiant energy. It transforms the mental substance by producing a particular thought movement. The rhythmical vibrations produced by Mantra regulate the unsteady vibrations of the five sheaths. It checks the natural tendency of objective thoughts of the mind. It helps the Sadhana Shakti and reinforces it. Sadhana Shakti is strengthened by Mantra-Shakti. Mantra awakens superhuman powers.

"Only the knowledge imparted by a Guru through his lips is powerful and useful; otherwise it becomes fruitless, weak and very painful." "*Siddhau visvasah prathamalakshanam*"—For success, firm belief is the first condition.

Develop the power of endurance (Titiksha); learn to bear happiness and misery evenly and to pass through all phases of life, all experiences.

The endurance of all pain and torture with patience and contentment means the exercise of a distinct force which spiritualizes the whole nature. The greater this force, the speedier the spiritual growth. Patience and faith should continue undiminished all through the Sadhana period.

Chitta-Shuddhi is purification of mind. Nadi Shuddhi is purification of Nadis. Bhuta-Shuddhi is purification of elements. Adhara-Shuddhi is purification of Adhara. If there is Shuddhi (purification), Siddhi (perfection) will come by itself. Siddhi is not possible without Shuddhi.

Humility is the highest of all virtues. You can destroy your egoism by developing this virtue alone. You can influence the whole world. You will become a magnet to attract the whole world. It must be genuine. Feigned humility is hypocrisy.

Control anger by practice of Kshama, Dhairya, patience and Nirabhimanata, absence of egoism.

When anger is controlled it will be transmuted into an energy by which you can move the whole world.

Anger is a modification of passion. If you can control lust, you have already controlled anger.

Drink a little water when you become angry. It will cool the brain and calm the excited, irritable nerves.

Count twenty, one by one. By the time you finish counting twenty, anger will subside.

Watch the small irritable impulse or thought-wave carefully. Then it will become easier for you to control anger. Take all precautions. Do not allow it to burst out and assume a wild form.

If you find it extremely difficult to control it, leave the place at once and walk for half an hour. Pray to God. Do Japa. Meditate. Meditation gives immense strength.

Very often depression comes in meditation in neophytes owing to the influence of Samskaras, influence of astral entities, evil spirits, bad company, cloudy days, bad stomach and loaded bowels. It must be quickly removed by cheerful thoughts, a brisk walk, singing His Name, and laughing, prayer, Pranayama, purgative and a dose of carminative mixture.

If you want to enter into Samadhi quickly, cut all connections with friends, relatives and others. Observe Akhanda Mowna. Live on milk alone. Plunge in meditation. Laziness and fickleness of mind are the two great obstacles in Yoga. Light Sattvic diet and Pranayamas will remove laziness. Do not overload the stomach. Walk briskly in the compound hither and thither for half an hour.

"Diseases are generated in one's body through the following causes, viz., sleeping in day-time, late vigil overnight, excess of sexual intercourse, moving in crowd, checking of urine and feces, taking of unwholesome food and laborious mental work. If a Yogi is affected by any disease due to these causes, he says that the disease is due to his Yogic practice. This is the first obstacle in yoga."

"Disease, mental inactivity, doubt, indifference, laziness, tendency to go after sense-enjoyments, stupor, false perception, non-attainment of concentration and falling away from that when attained on account of restlessness, are the obstructing distractions." (Yoga Sutras I-30).

If a practitioner is gloomy, depressed and weak, surely there is some error in his Sadhana. If aspirants themselves are gloomy and peevish how can they impart joy, peace and strength to others? A cheerful and ever-smiling countenance is a sure sign of spirituality and Divine life.

O emotional, enthusiastic young aspirants! Do not take the movements of rheumatic winds in the back from chronic lumbago for ascent of Kundalini. Do your Sadhana with patience, perseverance till you get Samadhi. Master every stage in Yoga. Do not take up any higher courses before you completely master the lower steps.

O impatient aspirant! Do not bother much about awakening Kundalini. Premature awakening is not desirable. Do your Sadhana and Tapas systematically and regularly. Just as the gardener who waters the trees daily gets the fruits when the proper time comes so also you will enjoy the fruits of your Sadhana when the time comes. Purify and steady the mind now. Purify the Nadis. Then Kundalini will be awakened spontaneously.

The aspirant, even though he would have awakened the Kundalini by some means, will not be benefited at all if he has not developed the necessary qualifications. It is not possible for him to feel, and manifest all the benefits of awakening Kundalini.

There are some developed souls who are in a state of Samadhi naturally from their very birth. They have not acquired this by any exertion in this birth. They are called born Siddhas. They have finished their Sadhana in their previous births.

By continence, devotion to Guru and steady practice, success comes in Yoga after a long time. The aspirant should always be patient and persevering.

"Svastika, Gomukha, Padma, Hamsa—these are the Brahmic postures (Asanas). Vira, Mayura, Vajra and Siddha Asanas are the Raudra postures. Yoni is the Sakta posture. Paschimottanasana is the Shaiva posture."

"Control over the five elements (Bhutas) may be gained by practicing Dharana on their respective seats in the body. The seat of earth extends from the foot to the knee; the seat of water extends from the knee to the navel; the seat of fire, from navel to the throat; the seat of air, from the throat to the region between the eyebrows; and the seat of Akasa from the eyebrows to Brahmarandhra." Nada is like a pure crystal extending from the Muladhara to Sahasrara Chakra. It is that which is spoken of as Brahman or Paramatman.

In the beginning of your practice, you may get jerks of hands, legs, trunk and whole body. Sometimes the jerks will be terrible. Do not be afraid. Do not be troubled. It is nothing. It is due to sudden muscular contraction from new Pranic influence. The jerks will pass off after some time. You will have to pass through these stages.

As soon as Kundalini is awakened for the first time, a Yogi gets these six experiences which last for a short time—Ananda (spiritual bliss), Kampana (tremor of the body and limbs), Utthana (rising from the ground), Ghurni (divine intoxication), Murccha (fainting) and Nidra (sleep). Good health, lightness of the body, shining complexion, not to be affected by the tips of thorns, to endure hunger and thirst, to eat and drink much and to fast for a long time, to endure heat and cold, and to have control over the five elements, are some other symptoms of Yogic life.

"Only a Yogi leading the life of a Brahmachari and observing a moderate and nutritious diet obtains perfection in the manipulation of Kundalini". (Ghe. Sam. III-12).

Many people are attracted to the practice of Pranayama and other Yogic exercises, as it is through Yoga that psychic healing, telepathy, thought-transference, and other great Siddhis are obtained. If they attain success, they should not remain there alone. The Goal of life is not 'healing' and 'Siddhis'. They should utilize their energy in attaining the Highest.

Those who can do telepathy, psychic healing, etc., use only the Prana in a different way. For producing different results, the same Prana must be utilized in a different method. You should know the technique to use this from a Guru. By long practice you also can do everything successfully.

A Yogi on the appearance of certain Siddhis thinks that he has achieved the highest goal. He may give up his further Sadhana through false contentment. The Yogi, who is bent upon getting the highest Samadhi, must reject Siddhis whenever they come. Siddhis are invitations from Devatas. Only by rejecting these Siddhis, one can attain success in Yoga. He who craves for Siddhis is a worldly-minded man. He is a very big householder. Those who crave for Siddhis will never get them. If a Yogic student is tempted to attain Siddhis, his further progress is seriously retarded. He has lost the way.

Do not stop Sadhana when you get a few glimpses and experiences. Continue the practice till you attain perfection. Do not stop the practice and move about in the world. Examples are not lacking. Numerous persons have been ruined. A glimpse cannot give you safety.

You can do nothing by a happy-go-lucky life. Stick to one place for three years. Draw a program of daily routine. Then follow to the very letter at any cost. Then you are sure to succeed.

There is no use of dilly-dallying hither and thither in search of a Guru. If you search for him, you will never get him. If you make yourself deserving by the practice of all preliminary qualifications, he will doubtless come to you. It is within the power of everybody to attain success in Yoga. What is wanted is sincere devotion, constant and steady Abhyasa.

Never allow sentiment to overcome you one way or other. Wisely utilize every condition for the uplift of the soul and Chitta Suddhi.

Unless you are prepared to give up all you have for the service of the Lord and mankind, you are quite unfit for the spiritual path.

You first separate yourself from the body; then you identify yourself with the mind and then you function on the mental plane. Through concentration, you rise above body-consciousness; through meditation you rise above mind; and finally through Samadhi, you reach the goal.

A Hatha Yogi brings down the Prana by Jalandhara Bandha; by Mula Bandha he checks the downward tendency of Apana; having accustomed himself to the practice of Asvini Mudra, he makes the Apana go upward with the mind intent on Kumbhaka. Through Uddiyana

Bandha, he forces the united Prana-Apana to enter the Sushumna Nadi along with Kundalini, and through Sakti Chalana Mudra, he takes Kundalini from Chakra to Chakra. By this procedure a Hatha Yogi makes conquest over Deha Adhyasa.

Eliminate fear altogether by constantly raising an opposite current of thought in the mind. Constantly and intently think of courage. Fear is a Vikara, unnatural, temporary modification on account of Avidya. When fear disappears, the attachment for the body goes away and then it is easy for you to go above body-consciousness.

Do not be carried away by name and fame (Khyati). Ignore all these trivial things. Be steady in your practice. Never stop Sadhana till the final beatitude is reached.

Just as the man who foolishly runs after two rabbits will not catch hold of any one of them, so also a meditator who runs after two conflicting thoughts will not get success in any one of the two thoughts. If he has divine thoughts for ten minutes and then worldly conflicting thoughts for the next ten minutes he will not succeed in getting at the Divine consciousness.

Several aspirants in the name of Tapasya neglect the body. All possible care should be taken to keep the body in a healthy condition. A Sadhaka should take more care than a worldly man because it is with this instrument that he has to reach the Goal. At the same time he must be quite unattached to the body and be prepared to give it up at any moment. That is the proper ideal.

As to the qualification for renunciation, a man should have attained perfect purity of mind, stability of intellect, discrimination, disgust towards sensual pleasures and a keen desire for freedom. Unless a man has attained these qualifications, renunciation of active duties of life does not produce the desired effect.

If you want Samadhi, you must know well the process of
Dhyana. If you want Dhyana, you must know accurately the
method of Dharana. If you want Dharana, you must know
perfectly the method of Pratyahara. If you want
Pratyahara, you must know Pranayama. If you want
Pranayama you must know Asana well. Before going to the
practice of Asana, you should have Yama and Niyama.
There is no use of jumping into Dhyana without having the
various preliminary practices.

Some aspirants, when they cannot get milk or ghee,
stop their Yogic practices. If you cannot get milk or ghee,
you will have to take a little more quantity of bread and Dal.
Dal is more nutritious than milk. It is very, very substantial.
Sadhakas should not develop any habit at all. Habit means
slavery. People of slavish mentality are absolutely unfit for
the spiritual path. They should not be affected at all even if
they are placed under the worst circumstances.

Vedantins use different methods for getting Laya,
viz., (1) Antahkarana Laya Chintana, (2) Pancha Bhuta Laya
Chintana and (3) Omkara Laya Chintana. In Antahkarana
Laya, you must think that the mind is merged in Buddhi;
Buddhi in Avyaktam; and Avyaktam in Brahman. In Pancha
Bhuta Laya, you must think that the earth gets merged in
water, water in fire; fire in air; air in Akasa; Akasa in
Avyaktam; and Avyaktam in Brahman. In Omkara Laya, you
must think that Visva gets merged in Virat (Virat in the
letter 'A'), Taijasa in Hiranyagarbha (Hiranyagarbha in the
letter 'U'), Prajna in Ishvara (Ishvara in the letter 'M'). Jiva
Sakshi gets merged in Ishvara Sakshi, Ishvara Sakshi in
Ardhamatra of Omkara. Thus you can go back to the
original source, Brahman, who is the Yoni for all minds and
Pancha Bhutas. Brahman alone remains.

Annamaya Kosha is the physical body (Sthula Sarira).
Pranamaya Kosha, Manomaya Kosha and Vijnanamaya

Kosha are in the astral body (Sukshma Sarira). Anandamaya Kosha belongs to the causal body (Karana Sarira). Pranamaya Kosha contains the five Karma Indriyas. Manomaya and Vijnanamaya Koshas contain the five Jnana Indriyas.

Priya, Moda and Pramoda are the attributes of Anandamaya Kosha. Hunger and thirst belong to Pranamaya Kosha. Birth and death belong to the Annamaya Kosha. Harsha and Soka (exhilaration and depression) belong to Manomaya Kosha. Passion, hunger, greed, Sankalpa and Vikalpa are Dharmas of the Manomaya Kosha. Sleep and Moha belong to Anandamaya Kosha. Kartritva (agency) and Bhoktritva (enjoyment) belong to Vijnanamaya Kosha.

In Manomaya Kosha, Iccha-Shakti is working. In Vijnanamaya Kosha, Jnana-Shakti is working. For other detailed information consult my book "Practice of Vedanta."

When Kundalini is awakened, it does not proceed at once to Sahasrara Chakra. By further Yogic practices, you will have to take it from Chakra to Chakra, one by one. Even after Kundalini has reached the Sahasrara it can drop to Muladhara Chakra. The Yogi can also stop it at a particular Chakra. When the Yogi is established in Samadhi, when he has attained Kaivalya, Kundalini will not come back to Muladhara.

The body will exist even after Kundalini has reached Sahasrara Chakra, but the Yogi will have no body-consciousness. It is only when Kaivalya is attained that the body becomes lifeless.

The Sadhakas should have a pure heart and should be free from Doshas. The Mantra should have been obtained from a great man. The Sadhaka should have faith in the Mantra. In this case, Japa alone is quite sufficient to awaken Kundalini.

Jnana Yoga, Mantra Yoga, Hatha Yoga, Raja Yoga and all other methods have the 8 steps, viz., Yama, Niyama, Asana, Pranayama, Pratyahara, Dharana, Dhyana, and Samadhi. These are not the exclusive property of Raja Yoga alone. These are necessary for all Sadhakas.

Young boys have no settled mind. Many have not the power of discrimination. Therefore young age is not suitable for advanced courses in Yoga.

Many other important doubts of the aspirants have been cleared in the text.

Some Practical Hints

The actual method of awakening the Kundalini Shakti and uniting Her with the Lord in the Sahasrara can only be learnt from a Guru. I give here a general outline of the Yogic practice that will enable the Sadhaka to realize the Chit.

The Jivatma in the subtle body, the receptacle of the five vital airs (Pancha Pranas), mind in its three aspects of Manas, Buddhi and Ahankara; the five organs of action (Karmendriyas); and the five organs of perception (Jnanendriyas), are united with the Kula-Kundalini. The Kandarpa or Kama Vayu in the Muladhara—a form of the Apana Vayu—is given a leftward revolution and the fire which is around Kundalini is kindled. By the Bija "Hung," and the heat of the fire thus kindled, the coiled and sleeping Kundalini is awakened. She who lay asleep around Svayambhu-linga, with her coils three circles and a half, dosing the entrance of the Brahmadvara, will on being roused, enter that door and move upwards, united with the Jivatma.

On this upward movement, Brahma, Savitri, Dakini-Shakti, the Devas, Bija and Vritti, are dissolved in the body of Kundalini. The Maheemandala or Prithvi is converted into the Bija "Lang," and is also merged in Her body. When Kundalini leaves the Muladhara, the lotus which, on the awakening of Kundalini, had opened and turned its flower upwards, again closes and hangs downwards. As Kundalini reaches the Svadhishthana-Chakra, that lotus opens out, and lifts its flower upwards. Upon the entrance of Kundalini, Mahavishnu, Mahalakshmi, Sarasvati, Rakini Shakti, Deva Matrikas and Vritti, Vaikunthadhama, Goloka, and the Deva and Devi residing therein are dissolved in the body of Kundalini. The Prithvi or earth Bija "Lang" is dissolved in Apah, and Apah converted into the Bija "Vang," remains in the body of Kundalini. When the Devi reaches the Manipura Chakra all that is in the Chakra merges in Her body. The Varuna Bija "Vang" is dissolved in fire, which remains in the body of the Devi as the Bija "Rang". This Chakra is called the Brahmagranthi (or knot of Brahma).

The piercing of this Chakra may involve considerable pain, physical disorder, and even disease. On this account, the directions of an experienced Guru are necessary, and therefore also other modes of Yoga have been recommended for those to whom they are applicable; for in such modes activity is provoked directly in the higher center and it is not necessary that the lower Chakras should be pierced. Kundalini next reaches the Anahata Chakra where all which is therein is merged in Her. The Bija of Tejas, "Rang" disappears in Vayu and Vayu converted into its Bija "Yang", merges into the body of Kundalini. This Chakra is known as Vishnugranthi (knot of Vishnu). Kundalini then ascends to the abode of Bharati (or Sarasvati) or the Vishuddha Chakra. Upon Her entrance,

Ardha-Narisvara Siva, Sakini, the sixteen vowels, Mantra, etc., are dissolved in the body of Kundalini. The Bija of Vayu, "Yang" is dissolved in Akasa, which itself being transformed into the Bija "Hang" is merged in the body of Kundalini. Piercing the Lalana Chakra, the Devi reaches the Ajna Chakra, where Parama Shiva, Siddha Kali, the Deva-Gana and all else therein are absorbed into Her body. The Bija of Akasa, "Hang" is merged in the Manas-Chakra and mind itself in the body of Kundalini. The Ajna Chakra is known as Rudra-granthi (or the knot of Rudra or Shiva). After this Chakra has been pierced, Kundalini, of Her own motion, unites with Paramasiva. As She proceeds upwards from the two-petaled lotus, the Niralamba Puri, Pranava Nada etc., are merged in Her.

The Kundalini then in her progress upwards, absorbs herself the twenty-four Tattvas commencing with the gross elements, and then unites Herself and becomes one with Paramasiva. The nectar, which flows from such union, floods the Kshudrabrahmanda or human body. It is then that the Sadhaka forgetful of all in this world is immersed in ineffable bliss.

Thereafter the Sadhaka, thinking of the Vayu Bija "Yang" as being in the left nostril, inhales through Ida, making Japa of the Bija sixteen times. Then closing both nostrils, he makes Japa of the Bija sixty-four times. He then thinks that the black "man of sin" (Papapurusha) in the left cavity of the abdomen is being dried up, and so thinking, he exhales through the right nostril Pingala, making Japa of the Bija thirty-two times. The Papapurusha should be thought of as an angry black man in the left side of the cavity of the abdomen, of the size of the thumb, with red beard and eyes, holding a sword and shield, with his head ever held low, the very image of all sins. The Sadhaka then meditating upon the red-colored Bija "Rang" in the

Manipura inhales, making sixteen Japas of the Bija, and then closes the nostrils, making sixty-four Japas. While making the Japa he thinks that the body of the man of sin is being burnt and reduced to ashes. He then exhales through the right nostril with thirty-two Japas. He then meditates upon the white Chandra Bija "Thang". He next inhales through Ida, making Japa of the Bija sixteen times, closes both nostrils with Japa done sixty-four times, and exhales through Pingala with thirty-two Japas. During inhalation, holding of breath and exhalation, he should consider that a new celestial body is being formed by the nectar (composed of all the letters of the alphabet, Matrika-varna) dropping from the moon. In a similar way with the Bija "Vang", the formation of the body is continued, and with the Bija "Lang" it is completed and strengthened. Lastly, with the Mantra "Soham", the Sadhaka leads the Jivatma into the heart. Thus Kundalini, who has enjoyed Her union with Paramashiva, sets out on her return journey the way she came. As she passes through each of the Chakras all that she has absorbed there from come out from herself and take their several places in the Chakra.

In this manner she again reaches the Muladhara, when all that is described to be in the Chakras are in the positions which they occupied before her awakening.

Spiritual Diary Month: _____

Questions	Date					
1. When did you get up from bed?						
2. How many hours did you sleep?						
3. How many Malas of Japa?						
4. How long in Kirtan?						
5. How many Pranayamas?						
6. How long did you perform Asanas?						
7. How long did you meditate in one Asana?						
8. How many Gita Slokas did you read or get by heart?						
9. How long in the company of the wise (Satsanga)?						
10. How many hours did you observe Mouna?						
11. How long in disinterested selfless service?						
12. How much did you give in charity?						
13. How many Mantras you						

wrote?						
14. How long did you practice physical exercise?						
15. How many lies did you tell and with what self-punishment?						
16. How many times and how long of anger and with what self-punishment?						
17. How many hours you spent in useless company?						
18. How many times you failed in Brahmacharya?						
19. How long in study of religious books?						
20. How many times you failed in the control of evil habits and with what self-punishment?						
21. How long you concentrated on your Ishta Devata (Saguna or Nirguna Dhyana)?						
22. How many days did you observe fast and vigil?						
23. Were you regular in your meditation?						
24. What virtue are you developing?						

25. What evil quality are you trying to eradicate?					
26. What Indriya is troubling you most?					
27. When did you go to bed?					

The Spiritual Diary

The Spiritual Diary is a whip for goading the mind towards righteousness and God. If you regularly maintain this diary you will get solace, peace of mind and make quick progress in the spiritual path. Maintain a daily diary and realize the marvelous results.

Prepare a statement of daily Spiritual Diary for every month as shown on the opposite page and verify whether you are progressing or not. If you want quick spiritual attainments, you should never neglect to record everything in your diary. To change the worldly nature it needs rigorous Sadhana. Apart from these questions you must also mention the following in the remarks column: —

1. The name of the Asanas.
2. The kind of meditation.
3. What books do you keep for Svadhyaya?
4. What is your special diet?
5. Do you keep a Japa Mala?
6. Have you got a separate meditation room?
7. How do you keep the meditation room?
8. Do you read Gita with meaning?

Do not be ashamed to mention your mistakes, vices and failures. This is meant for your own progress only. Do not waste your precious hours. It is enough that you have wasted so many years in idle-gossiping. Enough, enough of the troubles you had all these days in satisfying your senses. Do not say: —"from tomorrow I will be regular." That "tomorrow" is for the worthless worldly-minded fools. Be sincere and start doing Sadhana from this moment. Be sincere. Take out a copy of the Spiritual Diary and send it on to your Guru, who will guide you, remove all the obstacles in your Sadhana and give you further lessons.

Chapter Seven

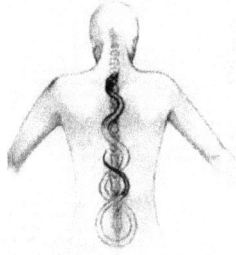

YOGA-KUNDALINI UPANISHAD

Introduction

The Yoga-Kundalini Upanishad is the eighty-sixth among the 108 Upanishads. It forms part of the Krishna Yajurveda. It deals with an exposition of Hatha and Lambika Yogas. It concludes with an account of the non-qualified Brahman. The Non-dual Brahman is the quest of all seekers. Though grouped among the minor Upanishads, the Yoga-Kundalini Upanishad is a very important work on Kundalini Yoga. It begins with an analysis of the nature of Chitta. It maintains that Samskaras and Vasanas on the one hand, and Prana, on the other, constitute the causes for the existence of Chitta. If Vasanas are controlled, Prana is automatically controlled. If Prana is controlled, the Vasanas are automatically controlled.

The Yoga-Kundalini Upanishad presents methods for the control of Prana. The Yogic student does not deal with Vasanas. He concerns himself with the techniques of controlling the Prana.

The three methods given in the Yoga-Kundalini Upanishad for the control of Prana are: Mitahara, Asana and Shakti-Chalana. These three methods are fully explained in the first chapter. Light, sweet and nutritious food forms the discipline of Mitahara. The Padmasana and the Vajrasana are two important Asanas used by the Yogic student. Shakti-Chalana is arousing the Kundalini and sending it to the crown of the head.

Kundalini can be aroused by a twofold practice. Saraswati Chalana and the restraint of Prana are the two practices. The rousing of the Saraswati Nadi is Saraswati Chalana.

The process, as described in the Yoga-Kundalini Upanishad, for arousing Kundalini is simple. When a person exhales, the Prana goes out 16 digits. In inhalation it goes in only 12 digits, thus losing 4. The Kundalini is aroused if one can inhale Prana for 16 digits. This is done by sitting in Padmasana and when the Prana is flowing through the left nostril, and lengthening inwards 4 digits more.

By means of this lengthened breath the Yogic student should manipulate the Saraswati Nadi and stir up the Kundalini Shakti with all his strength, from right to left, repeatedly. This process may extend to three quarters of an hour. All this has been briefly and yet comprehensively described in the Yoga-Kundalini Upanishad.

The most important result of shaking the Saraswati Nadi is that it cures the several diseases arising within the belly, and cleanses and purifies the system. After the practice of the Sahita Kumbhaka the Yogic student is initiated into the Kevala Kumbhaka. These two types of Kumbhaka bring about the complete restraint of the Prana. Suryabheda Kumbhaka, Ujjayi Kumbhaka, Sitali and Bhastrika are the four divisions of the Sahita Kumbhaka. Suryabheda Kumbhaka destroys the intestinal worms and the four kinds of evils caused by Vayu. Ujjayi purifies the body, removes diseases and increases the gastric fire. It also removes the heat caused in the head and the phlegm in the throat. Sitali cools the body. It destroys gulma, dyspepsia, pliha, consumption, bile, fever, thirst and poison. These forms of Sahita Kumbhaka purify and prepare the entire physiological organism for the arousal of the Kundalini Sakti and for the experience of the non-dual Brahman.

Apart from bringing a number of wholesome physiological changes, Bhastrika Kumbhaka pierces the three knots or the Granthis. The Yoga-Kundalini Upanishad then proceeds to prescribe the practice of the three Bandhas, for the Yogic student. The process by which the downward tendency of the Apana (breath) is forced up by the sphincter muscles of the anus is called the Mulabandha. By this Bandha, the Apana is raised up. It reaches the sphere of Agni or fire. Then the flame of the Agni grows long, being blown about by Vayu. In a heated state, Agni and Apana commingle with the Prana. This Agni is very fierce.

Through this fiery Agni, there arises in the body the fire that awakens and arouses the Kundalini, through its radiant heat. The aroused Kundalini makes a hissing noise, becomes erect and enters the hole of Brahmanadi. The Yogins practice this Mulabandha daily.

In this aim of arousing the Sarasvati Nadi and the Kundalini Shakti, the other two Bandhas, viz., Uddiyana Bandha and the Jalandhara Bandha, also play the most significant part.

After giving detailed knowledge of the techniques of the Bandhas, the Yoga-Kundalini Upanishad explains the number of obstacles the Yogic students encounter. It also gives the methods of overcoming these obstacles.

The causes of the diseases in the body are seven. 1. Sleeping during the daytime. 2. Late vigils overnight. 3. Excess of sexual intercourse. 4. Moving amidst crowds. 5. The effect of unwholesome food. 6. Checking of the discharge of urine and feces. 7. Laborious mental operations with the Prana.

The mistake that the Yogic student commits is that when diseases attack him, he erroneously attributes the diseases to his practice of Yoga. This is the first obstacle in Yoga.

The Yogic student begins to doubt as to the efficacy of the Yoga Sadhana. This is the second obstacle. Carelessness or a state of confusion is the third obstacle. Indifference or laziness is the fourth obstacle. Sleep is the fifth obstacle and the sixth is the attachment to sense-objects. The seventh obstacle is erroneous perception or delusion. The eighth is concern with worldly affairs. The ninth is want of faith. The tenth obstacle to Yoga practice is want of the necessary aptitude for grasping the Yoga truths.

Earnest spiritual aspirants should avoid all these obstacles by means of a close investigation and great deliberation. Further on, the Upanishads describe the process and the manner by which the Kundalini is roused and taken to the Sahasrara by piercing through the Granthis.

When the awakened Kundalini moves upwards, the shower of nectar flows copiously. The Yogi enjoys this which keeps him away from all sensual pleasures. The Yogi takes his stand upon the Inner Reality, the Atman. He enjoys the highest state of spiritual experience. He attains peace and is devoted only to the Atman.

By the whole process of the Kundalini Yoga Sadhana, the body of the Yogi attains very subtle state of the spiritual Consciousness. The Yogi who has attained to Samadhi experiences everything as Consciousness. The Yogi realizes the oneness of the macrocosm and the microcosm. Because, the Kundalini Shakti has reached the Sahasrara Kamala or the thousand-petaled lotus and has become united with Siva, the Yogi enjoys the highest Avastha. This is the final beatitude.

The Chakras are centers of Shakti as vital force. These are the centers of Prana Shakti manifested by Pranavayu in the living body.

Those aspirants, who aspire to arouse the Kundalini Shakti to enjoy the Bliss of Union of Siva and Shakti, through awakened Kundalini, and to gain the accompanying Powers or Siddhis, should practice Kundalini Yoga. To them, this Yoga-Kundalini Upanishad is of great importance. It equips them with a comprehensive knowledge of the methods and processes of the Kundalini Yoga in which the Khechari Mudra stands prominent.

The Kundalini Yogi seeks to obtain both Bhukti and Mukti. He attains liberation in and through the world. Jnana Yoga is the path of asceticism and liberation. Kundalini Yoga is the path of enjoyment and liberation.

The Hatha Yogi seeks a body which shall be as strong as steel, healthy, free from suffering and therefore, long-lived. Master of the body, the Yogi is the Master of life and death. His shining form enjoys the vitality of youth. He lives as long as he has the will to live and enjoys in the world of forms. His death is the death at will (Ichha-Mrityu). The Yogi should seek the guidance of an expert and skilled Guru.

The Serpent Power is the power which is the static support or Adhara of the whole body and all its moving Pranic forces. The polarity as it exists in, and as, the body is destroyed by Yoga, which disturbs the equilibrium of bodily consciousness, which consciousness is the result of the maintenance of these two poles.

In the human body the potential pole of Energy, which is the Supreme Power, is stirred to action. The Shakti is moved upward to unite with the Siva, the quiescent Consciousness in the Sahasrara.

By Pranayama and other Yogic processes the static Shakti is affected and becomes dynamic. When completely dynamic, when Kundalini unites with Siva in the Sahasrara, the polarization of the body gives way. The two poles are united in one and there is the state of consciousness called Samadhi. The polarization takes place in the Consciousness. The body actually continues to exist as an object of observation to others.

When the Kundalini ascends, the body of the Yogi is maintained by the nectar which flow, from the union of Siva and Shakti in Sahasrara. Glory to Mother Kundalini who, through Her Infinite Grace and Power, kindly leads the Sadhaka from Chakra to Chakra and illumines him and makes him realize his identity with the Supreme Brahman! The Yoga-Kundalini Upanishad attaches great importance to the search for and finding of right Guru. It insists upon revering the illumined Guru, as God. Guru is one who has full Self-illumination. He removes the veil of ignorance in the deluded individuals.

The number of realized Gurus may be less in this Kali Yuga when compared with the Satya Yuga, but they are always present to help the aspirants. They are always searching for the proper Adhikarins.

The Yoga-Kundalini Upanishad gives a list of the obstacles to Yoga practice. Some take to the practice of Yoga, and later on, when they come across some obstacles in the way, they do not know how to proceed further. They do not know how to obviate them. Many are the obstacles, dangers, snares and pitfalls on the spiritual path. Sadhakas may commit many mistakes on the path. A Guru, who has already trodden the path and reached the goal, is very necessary to guide them.

One more important thing, which you would find in many places in the Yoga-Kundalini Upanishad, is the Sushumna Nadi. You must have a complete knowledge of this Nadi.

Now, a word on Kundalini, the arousal of which is the immediate aim of the Kundalini Yoga. Kundalini, the serpent-power or mystic fire is the primordial energy or Shakti that lies dormant or sleeping in the Muladhara Chakra, the center of the body. It is called the serpentine or annular power on account of serpentine form. It is an electric fiery occult power, the great pristine force which underlies all organic and inorganic matter.

Chitta And The Control Of Prana

1. Chitta is the Subconscious mind. It is the mind-stuff. It is the storehouse of memory. Samskaras or impressions of actions are imbedded here. It is one of the four parts of Antahkarana or inner instruments, viz., mind, intellect, Chitta and Ahankara or ego.

2. Mind is formed out of wind. So, it is fleeting like the wind. Intellect is formed out of fire. Chitta is formed out of water. Ego is formed out of earth.

3. Chitta has two causes for its existence, viz., Vasanas or subtle desires and the vibration of Prana.

4. If one of them is controlled, the result is, both of them are controlled.

Mitahara, Asana And Shakti-Chalana

5. Of these two, viz., Prana and Vasanas, the student of Yoga should control Prana by moderate food (Mitahara), by Asanas or Yogic postures and thirdly by Shakti-Chalana.

6. O Gautama! I shall explain the nature of these three disciplines. Listen with rapt attention.

7. The Yogi should take sweet and nutritious food. He should fill half the stomach with food. He should drink water, one quarter of the stomach. He should leave the fourth quarter of the stomach unfilled in order to propitiate Lord Siva, the patron of the Yogins. This is moderation in diet.

The Padma And Vajra Asanas

8. Placing of the right foot on the left thigh and the left foot on the right thigh is Padmasana. This posture is the destroyer of all sins.

9. Placing one heel below the Muladhara and the other over it and sitting with the trunk, neck and head in one straight line is the adamantine posture or the Vajrasana. Mulakanda is the root of the Kanda, the genital organ.

The Rousing Of The Kundalini

10. A wise Yogi should take the Kundalini from the Muladhara to the Sahasrara or the thousand-petaled Lotus in the crown of the head. This process is called Shakti-Chalana.

11. The Kundalini should pass through the Svadhishthana Chakra, the Manipura Chakra in the navel, the Anahata Chakra in the heart, the Vishuddha Chakra in the throat, and the Ajna Chakra between the eyebrows or the Trikuti.

12. Two things are necessary for the practice of Shakti-Chalana. One is the Sarasvati Chalana and the other is the restraint of Prana or the breath.

The Sarasvati Chalana

13. Sarasvati Chalana is the rousing of the Sarasvati Nadi. Sarasvati Nadi is situated on the west of the navel among the fourteen Nadis. Sarasvati is called Arundhati. Literally, it means that which helps the performance of good actions.

14. Through this practice of Sarasvati Chalana and the restraint of the Prana, the Kundalini, which is spiral, becomes straightened.

15. The Kundalini is roused only by rousing the Sarasvati.

16. When Prana or the breath is passing through one's Ida or the left nostril, one should sit firmly in Padmasana and lengthen inwards 4 digits the Akasa of 12 digits. In exhalation Prana goes out 16 digits and in inhalation it goes in only 12 digits, thus losing 4. But if inhaled for 16 digits then the Kundalini is aroused.

17. The wise Yogi should bring Sarasvati Nadi by means of this lengthened breath and holding firmly together both the ribs near the navel by means of the forefinger and thumbs of both hands one hand on each side, should stir up Kundalini with all his strength, from right to left, again and again. This stirring may extend over a period of 48 minutes.

18. Then he should draw up a little when Kundalini finds its entry into Sushumna. This is the means by which the Kundalini enters the mouth of Sushumna.

19. Along with the Kundalini, Prana also enters of itself the Sushumna.

20. The Yogic student should also expand navel by compressing the neck. After this, by shaking Sarasvati, the

Prana is sent above to the chest. By the contraction of the neck, Prana goes above from the chest.

21. Sarasvati has sound in her womb. She should be thrown into vibration or shaken daily.

22. Merely by shaking Sarasvati one is cured of dropsy or Jalodara, Gulma (a disease of the stomach), Pliha (a disease of the spleen) and all other diseases rising within the belly.

Varieties Of Pranayama

23. Briefly, I will now describe to you Pranayama. Prana is the Vayu that moves in the body. The restraint of Prana within is known as Kumbhaka.

24. Kumbhaka is of two kinds, namely, Sahita and Kevala.

25. Till he gets Kevala, the Yogic student should practice Sahita.

26. There are four divisions or Bhedas. These divisions are: Surya, Ujjayi, Sitali and Bhastrika. Sahita Kumbhaka is the Kumbhaka associated with these four.

Suryabheda Kumbhaka

27. Select a place which is pure, beautiful and free from pebbles, thorns, etc. It should be of the length of a bow free from cold, fire and water. To this place, take a pure and pleasant seat which is neither too high nor too low. Upon it, sit in Padmasana. Now, shake or throw into vibration Sarasvati. Slowly inhale the breath from outside, through the right nostril, as long as this is comfortable, and exhale it through the left nostril. Exhale after purifying the skull by forcing the breath up. This destroys the four kinds of evils caused by Vayu. It destroys also the intestinal worms. This should be repeated often. It is called Suryabheda.

Ujjayi Kumbhaka

28. Close the mouth. Draw up slowly the breath through both the nostrils. Retain it in the space between the heart and the neck. Then exhale through the left nostril.

29. This removes both the heat caused in the head and the phlegm in the throat. It removes all diseases. It purifies the body and increases the gastric fire. It removes all the evils arising in the Nadis, Jalodara or dropsy, that is water in the belly, and Dhatus. The name for this Kumbhaka is Ujjayi. It can be practiced even when walking or standing.

Sitali Kumbhaka

30. Draw up the breath through the tongue with the hissing sound *Sa*. Retain it as before. Then slowly exhale through both the nostrils. This is called Sitali Kumbhaka.

31. Sitali Kumbhaka cools the body. It destroys gulma or the chronic dyspepsia, Pliha (a disease of the spleen), consumption, bile, fever, thirst and poison.

32. Sit in Padmasana with belly and neck erect. Close the mouth and exhale through the nostrils. Then inhale a little up to the neck so that the breath will fill the space, with noise, between the neck and skull. Then exhale in the same way and inhale often and often. Even as the bellows of a smith are moved stuffed within with air and then let out, so you should move the air within the body. When you get tired, inhale through the right nostril. If the belly is full of Vayu, press well the nostrils with all your fingers except the forefinger. Perform Kumbhaka and exhale through the left nostril.

33. This removes the inflammation of the throat. It increases the digestive gastric fire within. It enables one to know the Kundalini. It produces purity, removes sins, gives pleasure and happiness and destroys phlegm which is the bolt or obstacle to the door at the mouth of Brahmanadi or the Sushumna.

34. It pierces also the three Granthis or knots differentiated through the three modes of Nature or Gunas. The three Granthis or knots are Vishnu Granthi, Brahma Granthi and Rudra Granthi. This Kumbhaka is called Bhastrika. The Hatha Yogic students should especially practice this.

The Three Bandhas

35. The Yogic student should now practice the three Bandhas. The three Bandhas are: the Mula Bandha, the Uddiyana Bandha and the Jalandhara Bandha.

36. *Mula Bandha*: Apana (breath), which has a downward tendency, is forced up by the sphincter muscles of the anus. Mula Bandha is the name of this process.

37. When Apana is raised up and reaches the sphere of Agni (fire) then the flame of Agni grows long, being blown about by Vayu.

38. Then, in a heated state, Agni and Apana commingle with the Prana. This Agni is very fiery. Through this there arises in the body the fire that rouses the sleeping Kundalini through its heat.

39. Then this Kundalini makes a hissing noise. It becomes erect like a serpent beaten with a stick and enters the hole of Brahmanadi or the Sushumna. Therefore, the Yogins should practice daily Mulabandha often.

40. *The Uddiyana Bandha*: At the end of the Kumbhaka and at the beginning of expiration, Uddiyana Bandha should be performed. Because *Prana Uddiyate*, or

the *Prana* goes up the Sushumna in this Bandha, the Yogins call it Uddiyana.

41. Sit in the Vajrasana. Hold firmly the two toes by the two hands. Then press at the Kanda and at the places near the two ankles. Then gradually upbear the Tana or the thread or the Nadi which is on the western side first to Udara or the upper part of the abdomen above the navel, then to the heart and then to the neck. When the Prana reaches the Sandhi or the junction of the navel, slowly it removes the impurities and diseases in the navel. For this reason, this should be practiced frequently.

42. *The Jalandhara Bandha:* This should be practiced at the end of Puraka (after inhalation). This is of the form of contraction of the neck and is an impediment to the passage of Vayu (upwards).

43. The Prana goes through Brahmanadi on the western Tana in the middle, when the neck is contracted at once by bending downwards so that the chin may touch the breast. Assuming the posture as mentioned before, the Yogi should stir up Sarasvati and control Prana.

How Many Times Kumbhaka Should Be Practiced

44. On the first day, Kumbhaka should be practiced four times.

45. It should be done ten times, on the second day, and then five times separately.

46. On the third day, twenty times will be enough. Afterwards Kumbhaka should be practiced with the three Bandhas and with an increase of five times each day.

The Obstacles To The Practice Of Yoga And How To Overcome Them

47. Seven are the causes of the diseases in the body. Sleeping during the daytime is the first, late vigils overnight

is the second, excess of sexual intercourse the third, moving amidst crowds the fourth. The fifth cause is the effect of unwholesome food. The sixth is the checking of the discharge of urine and feces. The seventh is the laborious mental operation with Prana.

48. When attacked by such diseases, the Yogi who is afraid of them says, "My diseases have arisen from my practices of Yoga." Then he will discontinue this practice. This is the first obstacle to Yoga.

49. The second obstacle to Yoga is the doubt as to the efficacy of Yoga practice.

50. Third obstacle is carelessness or a state of confusion.

51. The fourth is indifference or laziness.

52. Sleep constitutes the fifth obstacle to Yoga practice.

53. The sixth is not leaving the objects of senses; the seventh is the erroneous perception or delusion.

54. The eighth is sensual objects or concern with worldly affairs. The ninth is want of faith. The tenth is non-aptitude for understanding of the truths of Yoga.

The Rousing Of The Kundalini

55. The intelligent practitioner of Yoga should, by means of close investigation and great deliberation, avoid these ten obstacles.

56. With the mind firmly fixed on the Truth, the practice of Pranayama should be performed daily. Then the mind takes its repose in the Sushumna. The Prana therefore never moves.

57. When the impurities of the mind are thus removed and Prana is absorbed in the Sushumna, one becomes a true Yogin.

58. When the accumulated impurity, clogging the Sushumna Nadi, is completely removed and the passage of vital air through the Sushumna is effected by performing Kevala Kumbhaka, the Yogin forcibly causes the Apana with the downward course to rise upwards by the contraction of the anus (Mula Bandha).

59. Thus raised up, the Apana mixes with Agni. Then they go up quickly to the seat of Prana. Then, Prana and Apana uniting with one another, go to Kundalini which is coiled up and asleep.

60. Heated by Agni and stirred up by Vayu, Kundalini stretches its body in the interior of the mouth of the Sushumna.

The Kundalini Reaches The Sahasrara By Piercing Through The Three Knots

61. The Kundalini pierces through the Brahmagranthi formed of Rajas. It flashes at once like lightning at the mouth of Sushumna.

62. Then Kundalini goes up at once through Vishnugranthi to the heart. Then it goes up through the Rudragranthi and above it to the middle of the eyebrows.

63. Having pierced this place, the Kundalini goes up to the Mandala (sphere) of the moon. It dries up the moisture produced by the moon in the Anahata Chakra which has sixteen petals.

64. Through the speed of Prana, when the blood is agitated, it becomes bile from its contact with the sun. Then it goes to the sphere of the moon. Here it becomes of the nature of pure phlegm.

65. When it flows there, how does the blood, which is very cold, become hot?

66. Since at the same time the intense white form of moon is rapidly heated. The agitated Kundalini moves upwards and the shower of nectar flows more copiously.

67. As a result of swallowing this, the Chitta of the Yogin is kept away from all sensual pleasures. The Yogin is exclusively absorbed in the Atma partaking of the sacrificial offering called nectar. He takes his stand in his own Self.

68. He enjoys this highest state. He becomes devoted to the Atman and attains peace.

The Dissolution Of Prana And Others

69. The Kundalini then goes to the seat of the Sahasrara. It gives up the eight forms of the Prakriti: earth, water, fire, air, ether, mind, intellect and egoism.

70. After clasping the eye, the mind, the Prana and the others in her embrace, the Kundalini goes to Siva and clasping Siva as well, dissolves herself in the Sahasrara.

71. Thus Rajas-Sukla or the seminal fluid, which rises up, goes to Siva along with Marut or the Vayu. Prana and Apana, which are always produced, become equal.

72. Prana flows in all things, big and small, describable or indescribable, as fire in gold. The breath also dissolves itself.

73. Born together of the same quality, the Prana and the Apana also dissolve themselves in the presence of Siva in the Sahasrara. Having reached an equipoised condition, they no longer go up or down.

74. Then the Yogi thrives with the Prana spread outward in the form of attenuated elements or in the mere remembrance of it, the mind having been reduced to the form of faint impressions and the speech having remained only in the form of recollection.

75. All the vital airs then spread themselves outright in his body even as gold in a crucible placed on fire.

Experiencing Everything As Consciousness During Samadhi

76. The body of the Yogi attains very subtle state of the pure Brahman. By causing the body made of the elements to be absorbed in a subtle state in the form of the Paramatman or the supreme Deity, the body of the Yogi gives up its impure corporal state.

77. That alone is the Truth underlying all things, which is released from the state of non-sentience and is devoid of impurities.

78. That alone which is of the nature of the Absolute Consciousness, which is of the character of the attribute "I" of all beings, the Brahman, the subtlest form of That alone is the Truth underlying all things.

79. The release from the notion that the Brahman is qualified, the delusion about the existence or non-existence of anything apart from the Brahman (which should be annihilated) and experience such as these that remain, there the Yogi should know as the Brahman. Simultaneously with the drawing of such knowledge of the form of the Atman, the liberation is attained by him.

80. When such is not the case, only all kinds of absurd and impossible notions arise. The rope-serpent and such other absurd notions, brought about by delusion take their rise. Absurd notions like the notion which men and women have, of silver, in the shell of the pearl oyster, arise.

81. The Yogi should realize the oneness of the Visvatman and others up to the Turiya. He should realize the oneness of the microcosm with the Virat Atman and others, up to the Turiya, of the macrocosm, also of the Linga with the Sutratman, of the Self with the unmanifested state, of the Atman manifested in one's Self with the Atman of Consciousness.

The Samadhi Yoga

82. The Kundalini Sakti is like a thread in the Lotus. It is resplendent. It is biting with its mouth, the upper end of its body, at the root of the Lotus, the Mulakanda or the Muladhara.

83. It is in contact with the hole of Brahmanadi of Sushumna, taking hold of its tail with its mouth.

84. Seated in Padmasana, if a person who has accustomed himself to the contraction of his anus (Mula Bandha), makes the Vayu go upwards with the mind intent on Kumbhaka, the Agni comes to the Svadhishthana flaming, owing to the blowing of Vayu.

85. From the blowing of Vayu and Agni, Kundalini pierces open the Brahmagranthi. It then pierces open the Vishnugranthi.

86. Then the Kundalini pierces the Rudragranthi. After that, it pierces all the six lotuses or the plexus. Then the Kundalini Sakti is happy with Siva in Sahasradala Kamala, the thousand-petaled lotus. This should be known as the highest Avastha or the state. This alone is the giver of final beatitude. Thus ends the first chapter.

The Khechari Vidya

1. Now, then, a description of the science called Khechari.

2. He who has duly mastered this science is freed from old age and death, in this world.

3. Knowing this science, O Sage, one who is subject to the pains of death, disease and old age, should make his mind firm and practice Khechari.

4. He who has gained a knowledge of the Khechari from books, from the exposition of the meaning of the same, and who has by recourse to its practice, gained a

mastery of this science, becomes the destroyer of old age, death and disease, in this world.

5. Such a master, one should approach for shelter. From all points of view, one should look upon him as his Guru.

6. The science of Khechari is not easily accessible. Its practice is not easily attainable. Its practice and Melana are not accomplished simultaneously. Literally, Melana is joining.

7. The key to this science of Khechari is kept a profound secret. The secret is revealed by adepts only at initiation.

8. They do not get Melana, who are bent only upon practice. O Brahman, only some get the practice after several births. But, even after hundred births, Melana is not obtained.

9. As a result of having undergone the practice for several births, some Yogis get the Melana in some future birth.

10. The Yogi attains the Siddhi mentioned in several books, when he gets this Melana from the mouth of the Guru.

11. The state of Siva freed from all rebirth, is achieved when the practitioner gets this Melana from the grasp of the significance presented in the books.

12. This science is, therefore, very difficult to master. Until he gets this science, the ascetic should wander over earth.

13. The ascetic has physical powers or Siddhis in his hand, the moment he obtains this science.

14. One should therefore regard as Achyuta or Vishnu, any person who imparts this Melana. He too should be regarded as Achyuta, who gives this science. He, who teaches the practice, should be regarded as Siva.

15. You have got the science from me. You should not reveal it to others. One, who knows this science, should practice it with all his efforts. Except to those who deserve it, he should give it to none.

16. One who is able to teach the Divine Yoga is the Guru. To the place where he lives, one should go. Then, learn from him the science of Khechari.

17. Taught well by him, one should at first practice it carefully. A person will then attain the Siddhi of Khechari, by means of this science.

18. One becomes the Lord of Khecharas or the Devas, by joining with Khechari Shakti (viz., Kundalini Shakti) by means of this science of Khechari. He lives amongst them, always.

The Khechari Mantra

19. Khechari contains the Bija or the seed-letter. Khechari Bija is spoken of as Agni encircled with water. It is the abode of the Devas or the Khecharas. The mastery of the Siddhi is obtained by this Yoga.

20. The ninth letter or Bija of Somamsa or the Moon face should be pronounced in the reverse order. Then consider it as the Supreme and its beginning as fifth. This is said to be Kuta (horns) of the several Bhinnas (or parts) of the moon.

21. Through the initiation of a Guru, this, which tends to the accomplishment of all Yogas, should be learnt.

22. One who recites this twelve times everyday will not get even in sleep that Maya or illusion which is born in his body and is the source of all vicious deeds.

23. To the one who recites these five lakhs of times with very great care, the science of Khechari will reveal itself. For him, all obstacles vanish. The Devas are pleased.

Without doubt, the destruction of the grayness of hair and wrinkles, Valipalita, will take place.

24. One who has acquired the great science should practice it constantly. Otherwise, he will not get any Siddhi in the path of Khechari.

25. If in this practice, one does not get this nectar-like science, he should get it in the beginning of Melana and recite it always. Otherwise, one who is without it never gets Siddhi.

26. No sooner one gets this science, than one should practice it. It is then that one will soon get the Siddhi.

27. The seven syllables HRIM, BHAM, SAM, PAM, PHAM, SAM and KSHAM constitute the Khechari Mantra.

The Cutting Of Frenum Lingui

28. A knower of the Atman, having drawn out the tongue from the root of the palate, should in accordance with the advice of his Guru, clear the impurities of the tongue for seven days.

29. He should take a sharp, oiled and cleansed knife, which resembles the leaf of the plant Snuhi, the milk-hedge plant, and should cut for the space of a hair, the frenum lingui. He should powder Saindhava or the rock salt and Pathya or the sea-salt and apply it to that place.

30. On the seventh day, he should again cut for the space of a hair. Thus, with great care, he should continue it always, for the span of six months.

31. The root of the tongue, fixed with veins, ceases to be in six months. Then the Yogi who knows timely action should encircle with cloth the tip of the tongue, the abode of Vag-Ishvari or the deity presiding over speech, and should draw it up.

The Tongue Reaches The Brahmarandhra

32. O Sage, again by daily drawing it up for six months, it comes as far as the middle of the eyebrows and obliquely up to the opening of the ears. By gradual practice, it goes up to the root of the chin.

33. Then, with ease it goes up to the end of the hair (of the head) in three years. It goes up obliquely to Sakha (some part below the skull) and downwards to the well of the throat.

34. It occupies Brahmarandhra, in another three years. Without doubt, it stops there. Crosswise it goes up to the top of the head and downwards to the well of the throat. Gradually it opens the great adamantine door in the head.

35. One should perform the six Angas or parts of the Khechari Bija Mantra by pronouncing it in six different intonations. In order to attain all the Siddhis, one should do this.

36. Karanyasa or the motions of the fingers and hands in the pronunciation of the Mantras should be done gradually. Karanyasa should never be done all at a time, because the body of one who does it all at once will soon decay. O best of the Sages, little by little it should be practiced.

37. One should, when the tongue goes to the Brahmarandhra through the outer path, place the tongue after moving the bolt of Brahma. The bolt of Brahma cannot be mastered by the Devas.

38. On doing this with the point of the finger for three years, the Yogi should make the tongue enter within. It enters the Brahmadvara or hole. On entering the Brahmadvara, one should practice well Mathana or churning.

39. Even without Mathana, some wise Yogis attain Siddhi. He also accomplishes it without Mathana, who is

versed in Khechari Mantra. One reaps the fruit soon by doing Japa and Mathana.

40. The Yogi should restrain his breath in his heart, by connecting a wire made of gold, silver or iron with the nostrils by means of a thread soaked in milk. Sitting in a convenient posture, with his eyes concentrated between his eyebrows, he should perform Mathana slowly.

41. The State of Mathana becomes natural like sleep in children, within six months. It is not advisable to do Mathana always. It should be done once only in every month.

The Urdhvakundalini Yoga

42. A Yogi should not revolve his tongue in the path. Twelve years of this practice will surely give the Siddhi to the Yogi. Then the Yogi perceives the entire universe in his body as not being different from the Atman.

43. O Chief of Kings, this path of the Urdhva Kundalini or the higher Kundalini, conquers the macrocosm. Here ends the second chapter.

Melana Mantra

1. *Melanamantra:* —Hrim, Bham, Sam, Sham, Pham, Sam and Ksham.

2. The Lotus-born Brahma said: Among new moon, the first day of the lunar fortnight and full moon, O Shankara, which is spoken of as the Mantra's sign? In the first day of lunar fortnight and during new moon and full moon days, it should be made firm. There is no other way or time.

Sense-Objects, Manas And Bandhana

3. Through passion, a person longs for an object. He is infatuated with passion for objects. These two one

should leave. The Niranjana or the Stainless should be sought after. All that one thinks is favorable to oneself should be abandoned.

4. The Yogin should keep the Manas in the midst of Shakti, and the Shakti in the midst of Manas. He should look into Manas by means of Manas. It is then that he leaves even the highest stage.

5. Manas alone is the Bindu. It is the cause of creation and preservation.

6. Like curd from milk, it is only through Manas that Bindu is produced. The organ of Manas is not that which is situated in the middle of Bandhana. Bandhana is there where Shakti is between the Sun and the Moon.

The Entry Into The Sukha-Mandala

7. The Yogi should stand in the seat of Bindu and close the nostrils, having known Sushumna and its Bheda or piercing and making the Vayu go in the middle.

8. After knowing Vayu, the above-mentioned Bindu and the Sattva-Prakriti as well as the six Chakras, one should enter the sphere of happiness, Sahasrara or the Sukha-Mandala.

The Six Chakras

9. There are six chakras. Muladhara is in the anus. Svadhishthana is near the genital organ. Manipuraka is in the navel. Anahata is in the heart.

10. The Vishuddhi Chakra is at the root of the neck. The sixth Chakra, the Ajna is in the head (between the two eyebrows).

11. After gaining a knowledge of these six Mandalas or spheres, one should enter the Sukhamandala, drawing up the Vayu and sending it upwards.

12. He becomes one with Brahmanda, the macrocosm, who practices thus the control of Vayu. He should master Vayu, Bindu, Chitta, and Chakra.

Abhyasa And Brahma Jnana

13. Through Samadhi alone, the Yogis attain the nectar of equality.

14. Without the practice of Yoga, the lamp of wisdom does not arise, even as the fire latent in the sacrificial wood does not appear without churning.

15. The fire in a vessel does not shed light outside. But, when the vessel is broken, its light appears without.

16. One's body is called the vessel. The seat of "That" is the light or the fire within. When, through the words of a Guru, the body is broken, the light of Brahmajnana becomes resplendent.

17. One crosses the subtle body and the ocean of Samsara, with the Guru as the helmsman, and through the affinities of Abhyasa.

The Four Kinds Of Vak

18. Sprouting in Para, Vak (power of speech) gives forth two leaves in Pasyanti, buds forth in Madhyama and blossoms in Vaikhari—that Vak, earlier described, reaches the stage of the absorption of sound, reversing the above order, viz., beginning with Vaikhari, etc.

19. Para, Pasyanti, Madhyama and Vaikhari, are the four kinds of Vak. Para is the highest of sounds. Vaikhari is the lowest of sounds.

20. Vak begins from the highest of sounds to the lowest, in evolution.

21. In involution it takes a reverse order in order to merge in Para or the highest subtle sound.

22. Anyone who thinks that the One who is the great Lord of that Vak, the undifferentiated, the Illuminator of that Vak is the Self—such a person who thinks over thus, is never effected by words, high or low, good or bad.

The Absorption In Paramatman

23. Through the absorption of their respective Upadhis or vehicles all these in turn are absorbed in the Pratyagatma—the three aspects of consciousness, Visva, Taijasa, and Prajna in man, the three, Virat, Hiranyagarbha, and Ishvara in the universe, the egg of the universe, the egg of man and the seven worlds.

24. Heated by the fire of Jnana, the egg is absorbed with its Karana or cause, into Paramatman or the universal Self. It becomes one with Parabrahman.

25. It is then neither steadiness nor depth, neither light nor darkness, neither describable nor distinguishable. That alone remains which is the Be-ness or the Sat.

The Essential Nature Of Man

26. Like a light in a vessel, the Atman is within the body—thus one should think.

27. Atman is of the dimensions of a thumb. It is a light without smoke. It is without form. It is shining within the body. It is undifferentiable and immortal.

28. The first three aspects of consciousness refer to the gross, subtle and Karana bodies of man. The second three aspects of consciousness refer to the three bodies of the universe.

29. In his formation, man is and appears as an egg, even as the universe is and appears as an egg.

30. During the states of waking, dreaming and dreamless sleep, the Vijnana Atma which dwells in this body is deluded by Maya.

31. But, after many births, owing to the effect of good Karma, it wishes to attain its own essential state.

32. The enquiry sets in. Who am I? How has this stain of mundane existence come to me? In the dreamless sleep what becomes of me who am engaged in business during both the states, waking and dreaming?

33. The Chidabhasa is the result of non-wisdom. It is burnt by the wise thoughts, even as a bale of cotton is burnt by fire, and also by its own supreme illumination.

34. The burning of the outer body is no burning at all.

35. Pratyagatma is in the Dahara (Akasa or the ether of the heart). It obtains, when the worldly wisdom is destroyed, Vijnana, and diffuses itself everywhere and in an instant burns the two sheaths, Vijnanamaya and Manomaya. Then, it is He Himself that shines always within. It shines like a light within a vessel.

36. Till sleep and till death, the Muni who contemplates thus should be known as a Jivanmukta.

Videha Mukti

37. He has done what ought to be done. Therefore, he is a fortunate person.

38. Such a person attains Videhamukti, having given up even the state of Jivanmukti.

39. No sooner the body wears off, than he obtains the emancipation in a disembodied state, Videhamukti. The state, as if of moving in the air, he gains.

Non-Dual Brahman

40. After that, That alone remains. That is the soundless, the touchless, the formless and the deathless.

41. That is the Rasa or the Essence. It is eternal and odorless. It is greater than the great; it has neither

beginning nor end. It is the permanent, the stainless and the decayless. Thus ends the Yoga-Kundalini Upanishad.

Kundalini Yoga

The Yogin who works for liberation does so through Kundalini Yoga which gives both enjoyment and liberation. At every center to which he rouses Kundalini he experiences special form of bliss and gains special powers. Carrying Her to Siva at his cerebral center, he enjoys the Supreme bliss which in its nature is that of Liberation and which when established in permanence is Liberation itself on the loosening of spirit and body.

Energy (Sakti) polarizes itself into two forms namely, static or potential (Kundalini) dynamic (the working forces of the body as Prana). Behind all activity there is a static background. This static center in the human body is the center serpent-power in the Muladhara (root support).

This static Sakti is affected by Pranayama and other Yogic processes and becomes dynamic. Thus when completely dynamic that is when Kundalini unites with Siva in the Sahasrara the polarization of the body gives way. The two poles are united in one and there is the state of consciousness called Samadhi. The polarization, of course, takes place in consciousness. The body actually continues to exist as an object of observation to others. It continues its organic life. But man's consciousness of his body and all other objects, is withdrawn because the mind has ceased so far as his consciousness is concerned, the function having been withdrawn into its ground which is Consciousness.

When awakened, Kundalini Sakti ceases to be a static power which sustains the world-consciousness, the content of which is held only so long as she sleeps; and when once set in movement Kundalini is drawn to that other static center in the Thousand-petaled Lotus (Sahasrara) to attain union with the Siva Consciousness or the consciousness of ecstasy beyond the world of forms. When Kundalini sleeps man is awake to this world. When she wakes he sleeps i.e. loses all consciousness of the world and enters the causal body. In Yoga he passes beyond to formless consciousness.

Pranayama for Awakening Kundalini: When you practice the following, concentrate on the Muladhara Chakra at the base of the spinal column which is triangular in form and which is the seat of the Kundalini Sakti. Close the right nostril with your right thumb. Inhale through the left nostril till you count 3 Oms slowly. Imagine that you are drawing the Prana with the atmospheric air. Then close the left nostril with your little and ring fingers of the right hand. Then retain the breath for 12 Oms. Send the current down the spinal column straight into the triangular lotus, the Muladhara Chakra. Imagine that the nerve-current is striking against the Lotus and awakening the Kundalini. Then slowly exhale through the right nostril counting 6 Oms. Repeat the process from the right nostril as stated above using the same units and having the same imagination and feeling. This Pranayama will awaken the Kundalini quickly. Do it 3 times in the morning and 3 times in the evening. Increase the number and time gradually and cautiously according to your strength and capacity. In this Pranayama concentration on the Muladhara Chakra is the important thing, Kundalini will be awakened quickly if the degree of concentration is intense and if the Pranayama is practiced regularly.

Kundalini Pranayama

In this Pranayama, the Bhavana is more important than the ratio between Puraka, Kumbhaka and Rechaka. Sit in Padma or Siddha Asana facing the East or the North. After mentally prostrating to the lotus-feet of the Sat-guru and reciting Stotras in praise of God and Guru, commence doing this Pranayama which will easily lead to the awakening of the Kundalini.

Inhale deeply without making any sound. As you inhale, feel that the Kundalini lying dormant in the Muladhara Chakra is awakened and is going up from Chakra to Chakra. At the conclusion of the Puraka, have the Bhavana that the Kundalini has reached the Sahasrara. The more vivid the visualization of Chakra after Chakra, the more rapid will be your progress in this Sadhana.

Retain the breath for a short while. Repeat the Pranava or your Ishta Mantra. Concentrate on the Sahasrara Chakra. Feel that by the Grace of Mother Kundalini, the darkness of ignorance enveloping your soul has been dispelled. Feel that your whole being is pervaded by light, power and wisdom.

Slowly exhale now. And, as you exhale feel that the Kundalini Sakti is gradually descending from the Sahasrara and from Chakra to Chakra, to the Muladhara Chakra.
Now begin the process again.

It is impossible to extol this wonderful Pranayama adequately. It is the magic wand for attaining perfection very quickly. Even a few days' practice will convince you of its remarkable glory. Start from today, this very moment. May God bless you with joy, bliss and immortality.

Lambika Yoga

Practice of Khechari Mudra is Lambika Yoga. The technique of the Mudra is explained below. He who practices this Mudra will have neither hunger nor thirst. He can walk in the sky. This Yoga is beset with difficulties.

This is a very difficult Yoga. It has to be learnt under a developed Yogi Guru who has practiced this Yoga for a long time and attained full success.

It is kept secret by Yogis. It confers great Siddhis or powers. It is a great help to control the mind. He, who has attained success in this Mudra, will have neither hunger nor thirst. He can control his Prana quite easily.

Khechari Mudra, Yoni Mudra or Shanmukhi Mudra, Sambhavi Mudra, Asvini Mudra, Maha Mudra and Yoga Mudra are the important Mudras. Among these Mudras, Khechari Mudra is the foremost. It is the king of the Mudras. Mudra means a seal. It puts a seal to the mind and Prana. Mind and Prana come under the control of a Yogi. Khechari Mudra consists of two important Kriyas viz., Chhedan and Dohan.

The lower part of the front portion of the tongue, the frenum lingua, is cut to the extent of a hair's breadth with a sharp knife once in a week. Afterwards powder of turmeric is dusted over it. This is continued for some months. This is Chhedan.

Afterwards the Yogic student applies butter to the tongue and lengthens it daily. He draws the tongue in such a way that it is similar to the process of milking the udder of a cow. This is Dohan.

When the tongue is sufficiently long (it should touch the tip of the nose) the student folds it, takes it back and closes the posterior portion of the nostrils. Now he sits and meditates. The breath stops completely. For some the cutting and the lengthening of the tongue is not necessary. They are born with a long tongue.

He who has attained perfection in this Mudra becomes a walker in the sky. Queen Chudala had this Siddhi or power.

He who has purity and other divine virtues, who is free from desire, greed and lust, who is endowed with dispassion, discrimination and strong aspiration or longing for liberation will be benefited by the practice of this Mudra. The Mudra helps the Yogi to get himself buried underneath the ground.

Yoga — I

Yoga is a perfect practical system of self-culture. Yoga is an exact science. It aims at the harmonious development of the body, the mind and the soul. Yoga is the turning away of the senses from the objective universe and the concentration of the mind within. Yoga is eternal life in the soul or spirit. Yoga aims at controlling the mind and its modifications. The path of Yoga is an inner path whose gateway is your heart.

Yoga is the discipline of the mind, senses and physical body. Yoga helps in the co-ordination and control of the subtle forces within the body. Yoga brings in perfection, peace and everlasting happiness. Yoga can help you in your business and in your daily life. You can have calmness of mind at all times by the practice of Yoga. You can have restful sleep. You can have increased energy, vigor, vitality, longevity and a high standard of health. Yoga transmutes animal nature into divine nature and raises you to the pinnacle of divine glory and splendor.

The practice of Yoga will help you to control the emotions and passions and will give you power to resist temptations and to remove the disturbing elements from the mind. It will enable you to keep a balanced mind always and remove fatigue. It will confer on you serenity, calmness and wonderful concentration. It will enable you to hold communion with the Lord and thus attain the *summum bonum* of existence.

If you want to attain success in Yoga, you will have to abandon all worldly enjoyments and practice Tapas and Brahmacharya. You will have to control the mind skillfully and tactfully. You will have to use judicious and intelligent methods to curb it. If you use force, it will become more turbulent and mischievous. It cannot be controlled by force. It will jump and drift away more and more. Those who attempt to control the mind by force are like those who endeavor to bind a furious elephant with a thin silken thread.

A Guru or preceptor is indispensable for the practice of Yoga. The aspirant in the path of Yoga should be humble, simple, gentle, refined, tolerant, merciful and kind. If you have a curiosity to get psychic powers you cannot have success in Yoga. Yoga does not consist in sitting cross-legged for six hours or stopping the pulse or beating of the heart or getting oneself buried underneath the ground for a week or a month.

Self-sufficiency, impertinence, pride, luxury, name, fame, self-assertive nature, obstinacy, idea of superiority, sensual desires, evil company, laziness, overeating, overwork, too much mixing and too much talking are some of the obstacles in the path of Yoga. Admit your faults freely. When you are free from all these evil traits, Samadhi or union will come by itself.

Practice Yama and Niyama. Sit comfortably in Padma or Siddhasana. Restrain the breath. Withdraw the senses. Control the thoughts. Concentrate. Meditate and attain Asamprajnata or Nirvikalpa Samadhi (union with the Supreme Self). May you shine as a brilliant Yogi by the practice of Yoga. May you enjoy the bliss of eternity.

Yoga — II

Yoga is primarily a process of self-culture. Its aim is the attainment of spiritual perfection or Self-realization. The process of Yoga pertains to the control of the physical organs, the breath, the mind and the senses.

Practice of Yoga bestows a rich and full life. It is, in fact, the science of living a pure and healthy life.

Practice of self-restraint, mental equipoise, truthfulness, compassion, purity and selflessness constitutes the process of Yoga.

Practice of Asana, Pranayama, Bandha and Mudra also constitutes the process of Yoga.

A nation composed of physically strong and mentally healthy people can surely be great.

Physical culture should start at an early age. Both body and mind should be trained. Exercises should provide both recreation and physical and mental development. Asanas keep the muscles supple, the spine elastic, develop mental faculties, lung capacity, strengthen the internal organs and bestow longevity.

Sirshasana develops the brain, confers good memory and improves eyesight and hearing capacity through extra circulation of blood in the brain box.

Sarvangasana develops the thyroid gland, strengthens the lungs and the heart, and makes the spine elastic.

Bhujangasana, Salabhasana and Dhanurasana increase the peristaltic movement of the bowels, remove constipation and cure the diseases of the abdomen.

Viparitakarani Mudra and Paschimottanasana tone up the pelvic muscles and the pelvic organs. They improve the digestive system. Agnisara Kriya, Uddiyana Bandha and Mayurasana also help digestion and give good appetite.

Ardha-matsyendrasana is good for appetite. Ardha-matsyendrasana is good for the liver and the spleen.

Rolling from side to side in Dhanurasana gives very good abdominal massage. Matsyasana is good for the development of the lungs, the brain and the eyes; it also strengthens the upper part of the spine. Savasana relaxes the body and the mind and gives perfect poise and rest. Women and children (above seven years) are not exempted from practicing Asanas.

Every Asana should be practiced only for a minute or two, but the period could be gradually extended to a limited duration as per the advice of a competent teacher. Pranayama bestows vigor, vitality and longevity. It develops the lungs and strengthens the muscles of the chest.

First practice deep inhalation and exhalation. Then try to hold the breath as far as it is comfortably possible. Practice a few rounds of deep breathing in the early hours of the morning.

In winter practice Bhastrika Pranayama and in summer Sitali and Sitkari.

Mild practice Of Pranayama needs no dietetic regulation or any particular condition of living.

Never exert yourself. Use your common sense. If you find any substantial benefit, continue your practice. If there is any discomfort, discontinue the practice and seek proper guidance.

Withdraw the mind from the external objects and try to fix your attention on a particular object or subject. Concentrate on the symbol of Om or on the picture of an Avatara or a saint.

Meditate on the divine qualities of auspiciousness, holiness, peace, sanctity, grace, equanimity, nobility, sincerity and selflessness. Try to cultivate these qualifies in your day-to-day life. Speak the truth always. Be kind-hearted.

Live the life of detachment and egolessness. Try to control your emotions. Try to restrain your impulses. Do not be domineering. Be humble, polite and courteous. Do not be jealous of another's prosperity. Do not be pessimistic. Do not try to become prosperous or famous at the expense of others.

Analyze your motives. Scrutinize your thoughts. Enquire into the nature of things. Do not run after the false glitter of the world. Restrain yourself. Forego personal comforts and luxuries if thereby you could be of some help to another. Always remember your essential, divine nature. This is the process of Yoga.

Ideal Yoga

Some Yogic students think that only he who can fly in the air, walk on the water, and do such other miracles, can be called a Yogi. It is a sad mistake. To be peaceful, to be calm, to radiate joy, to have an intense aspiration to realize God, to have the spirit of service and devotion, to be self-controlled—this is real Yoga. Flying in the air is not yoga. Why should one aspire to fly like a bird after attaining the human birth? You must have a willing heart to serve everybody and a desire to possess all divine virtues. This is Yoga.

Your ideal should be to be good, and to do good. Be ever willing to share what you have with others.

You should have a knowledge of the scriptures, devotion to your preceptor, saints and sages. Even Nirvikalpa Samadhi is not necessary. Why do you want to get yourself merged in the Absolute? Have a small veil of individuality and serve here as Nityasiddhas. Possess divine qualities and move as a divine being on this earth. Aspire not for powers. Powers will come by themselves. Possess all noble virtues. Be free from hatred and malice. Elevate others by your own example.

Spread the message of the Rishis. Lead a righteous life. Speak the truth. Worship mother as God, father as God, teacher as God and guest as God. Give; but give with modesty. Give with goodwill. Give with love.

There is one eternal Atma, one universal Consciousness that dwells in the hearts of all.

Realize this through aspiration, renunciation, concentration, and purification.

Control anger. Do not get irritated through misunderstanding. Try to understand everybody. Understand the feelings of others. Bear insult. Bear injury. Be ever intent on the welfare of all—*Sarvabhutahite ratah*. You should practice these—not merely study the Brahmasutras and the Upanishads. The Upanishads should come from your heart through purification, through Service.

Selfless service is the highest thing on this earth. Service will make you divine. Service is divine life. Service is eternal life in God. Service will give you Cosmic Consciousness—Service that is selfless, without attachment. But nobody wants to serve! Everybody wants to be served by others. You will have to kill the ego. You will have to pulverize it, make it a powder. You will have to extract oil from your bones and burn it for six months. Such is the toil, as it were, to progress in the path of self-realization.

Be good; do good. This is the essence of the teachings of all scriptures and prophets of the world. Those who want inner life are very few. All are thirsting for happiness, but they do not know where they can get happiness. They search for it in wealth and material possessions. Maya is clever. She never allows people to taste the bliss of an inner life in the Atman. Deluded by her power, man thinks that there is no transcendental realm, that there is nothing beyond the senses. "Eat, drink and be merry," this has become the motto of life. The path to the realm of God is open only to those who have got the Divine Grace.

May you all know the true import of Yoga, and base your life on selfless service to humanity with Atma Bhava, and the development of all divine virtues. May you all have sustained aspiration. Practice deep meditation and attain Self-realization. May you all shine as Nityasiddhas, radiating joy and peace all round.

Ten Commandments For Yoga-Students

1. Practice Asanas and Pranayama in the early morning or three hours after food.

2. Offer prayers to Guru and God before commencing the practice.

3. Take Sattvic food, avoid hot, pungent, sour articles of food and stimulants, like tea, coffee, etc.

4. Keep a clean room under lock and key; let it be well-ventilated, cool, free from insects and from other sources of disturbance.

5. Observe strict Brahmacharya; avoid unnecessary talks.

6. Reduce your wants. Develop contentment.

7. Take bath before the practice; if that is not possible, have a wash before and bath at least half an hour after the practice.

8. Sit facing East or North.

9. Be regular and systematic in your practice.

10. Obey your Guru implicitly in all respects.

Yoga And Its Consummation

Yoga is the art of uniting the individual soul with the Supreme Soul, of uniting the Kundalini Sakti lying dormant in the Muladhara Chakra with Siva in the Sahasrara Chakra. By convention, all practices that help the attainment of this goal are also called Yoga.

Vedanta says that the individual soul is enveloped by five sheaths—Annamaya Kosha (the gross body), Pranamaya Kosha (vital sheath), Manomaya Kosha (the mind), Vijnanamaya Kosha (the intellect), and Anandamaya Kosha (the bliss-sheath or the ignorance that immediately veils the Self), and that the goal of life, viz., Self-realization is attained by negating the five sheaths and piercing the veil of ignorance.

When do we regard a particular part or organ of the body as perfectly healthy? When we are not made aware of that organ. The ear is in perfect health when we are not aware that that organ exists; if there is pain we are conscious of its presence. In order to transcend the five sheaths, therefore, they must all be free from afflictions. Yoga helps you to do that.

The purificatory Kriyas of Hatha Yoga and Asanas ensure health of the body and free it from ailments. Pranayama revitalizes the vital sheath. Pratyahara (withdrawal of the rays of the mind and restraining them from flowing outwards) and Dharana (concentration) strengthen the mind. Meditation brings about a happy blending of the intellect and intuition; and the Yogi's intelligence becomes intuitive. Samadhi illumines the soul and reveals the Self, by piercing the veil of ignorance. This is Yoga, the perfect system of all-round self-culture.

But no one can embark on this noble enterprise without preparing the vessel. Yama-Niyama or the canons of right conduct, ensure this. One who has not controlled his senses, who is not truthful, kind, compassionate and pure, cannot make any progress in Sadhana. Energy leaks out through all the avenues of his body. His vital sheath is debilitated. His mind is completely extroverted. His intellect is dull. His soul is enveloped in dense darkness. Meditation for such a man is only a dream. Therefore I insist on all spiritual aspirants that they should: —

1. Engage themselves in Nishkama Karma Yoga, for self-purification and cultivation of virtues; and

2. Practice as much Japa as possible, in order to earn His Grace.

These two—Karma Yoga and Bhakti Yoga—cannot be overemphasized.

Once the senses are controlled, and the heart purified, control of mind, concentration of its rays, and meditation become very easy. The aspirant would do well to remember the two great watchwords of Sadhana—

(a) Abhyasa (unrelenting, intense, unbroken, regular and systematic practice),

(b) Vairagya (dispassion, aversion to all sensual enjoyments, non-attachment to objects of senses).

To the extent to which the aspirant grows in these two, to that extent will his mind *want to meditate*. There will be joy in meditation. The mind will look forward to the period of meditation. When this condition becomes intense, then the mind will be in a constant state of meditation. As your hands are engaged in the work of the day, the mind will be blissfully detached from the world, peacefully witnessing—Sakshi-Bhava—the play of the senses and the sense-objects. When you are established in this state, you are a perfected Yogi. You have only to sit and close your eyes; you will instantly transcend the five sheaths and merge in the Supreme Soul. Your actions will be in tune with the Divine Will. You will have the superhuman powers of intellect, mind and body. You will never be tired, dull or depressed. Your words will have life-transforming power. Your heart will be full of compassion and love for humanity, and all humanity will be drawn towards you. You will become a spiritual magnet. You will shine as a Yogi, sage and Jivanmukta. You are liberated. This is the Goal.

May God bless you.

The Gradational Ascent Of The Mind

The Chakras are centers of Shakti as vital force—in other words, these are centers of Pranashakti manifested by Pranavayu in the living body, the presiding Devatas of which are the names for the Universal Consciousness as it manifests in the form of these centers. The Chakras are not perceptible in the gross senses. Even if they were perceptible in the living body, which they help to organize, they disappear with the disintegration of organism at death.

Purity of mind leads to perfection in Yoga. Regulate your conduct when you deal with others. Have no feeling of jealousy towards others. Be compassionate. Do not hate sinners. Be kind to all. Success in Yoga will be rapid if you put your maximum energy in your Yoga practice. You must have a keen longing for liberation and intense Vairagya also. You must be sincere and earnest. Intense and constant meditation is necessary for entering into Samadhi. The mind of a worldly man with base desires and passions moves in the Muladhara and Svadhishthana Chakras or centers situated near the anus and the reproductive organ respectively.

If one's mind becomes purified the mind rises to the Manipura Chakra or the center in the navel and experiences some power and joy.

If the mind becomes more purified, it rises to the Anahata Chakra or center in the heart, experiences bliss and visualizes the effulgent form of the Ishta Devata or the tutelary deity.

When the mind gets highly purified, the meditation and devotion become intense and profound, the mind rises to Vishuddha Chakra or the center in the throat and experiences more and more powers and bliss. Even when the mind has reached this center, there is possibility for it to come down to the lower centers.

When the Yogi reaches the Ajna Chakra or the center between the two eyebrows he attains Samadhi and realizes the supreme Self or Brahman. There is a slight sense of separateness between the devotee and Brahman.

If he reaches the spiritual center in the brain, the Sahasrara Chakra, the thousand-petaled lotus the Yogi attains Nirvikalpa Samadhi or superconscious state—He becomes one with the non-dual Brahman. All sense of separateness dissolves. This is the highest plane of consciousness or Supreme Asamprajnata Samadhi. Kundalini unites with Siva.

The Yogi may come down to the center in the throat to give instructions to the students and do good to others (Lokasamgraha).

Experiences On Awakening Of Kundalini

During meditation you behold divine visions, experience divine smell, divine taste, divine touch, hear divine Anahata Sounds. You receive instructions from God. These indicate that the Kundalini Shakti has been awakened. When there is throbbing in Muladhara, when hair stands on its root, when Uddiyana, Jalandhara and Mulabandha come involuntarily, know that Kundalini has awakened.

When the breath stops without any effort, when Kevala Kumbhaka comes by itself without any exertion, know that Kundalini Shakti has become active. When you feel currents of Prana rising up to the Sahasrara, when you experience bliss, when you repeat Om automatically, when there are no thoughts of the world in the mind, know that Kundalini Shakti has awakened.

When, in your meditation, the eyes become fixed on Trikuti, the middle of the eyebrows, when the Sambhavi Mudra operates, know that Kundalini Shakti has become active. When you feel vibrations of Prana in different parts inside your body, when you experience jerks like the shocks of electricity, know that Kundalini has become active. During meditation when you feel as if there is no body, when your eyelids become closed and do not open in spite of your exertion, when electric-like currents flow up and down the nerves, know that Kundalini has awakened.

When you meditate, when you get inspiration and insight, when the nature unfolds its secrets to you, all doubts disappear, you understand clearly the meaning of the Vedic texts, know that Kundalini has become active. When your body becomes light like air, when you possess inexhaustible energy for work, know that Kundalini has become active.

When you get divine intoxication, when you develop power of oration, know that Kundalini has awakened. When you involuntarily perform different Asanas or poses of Yoga without the least pain or fatigue, know that Kundalini has become active. When you compose beautiful sublime hymns and poetry involuntarily, know that Kundalini has become active.

The Quintessence Of Yoga

Yoga is union with the infinite through meditation and Samadhi.

A Yogi is freed from Karma or the law of cause and effect, from births and deaths and from the trammels of mind and flesh.

The Yogi has perfect control over his life forces and mind. He can dematerialize at will.

The Yogi practices discipline of body and mind. He has control over his body and mind. He meditates on Om.

Yoga illumines, renovates and helps the Yogi to attain the highest point of perfection.

If one awakens his superconsciousness, there will be no problems at all. There will be only love, peace, harmony, unity and happiness in this world.

Practice Yoga To Prolong Life

The practice of Yoga lessens and prevents the decay of tissues, by increasing the life force, and fills the system with abundant energy.

By the practice of Yoga the blood is charged with abundant oxygen. The brain and spinal centers are rejuvenated.

By the practice of Yoga, the accumulation of venous blood is stopped. The body is filled with abundant energy. The brain-centers and the spinal cord are strengthened and renovated. Memory is improved. Intellect is sharpened. Intuition is developed.

How can one who does not know his own body hope to achieve success in Yoga? First have a strong, firm and healthy body through the practice of Hatha Yoga and then take to Raja Yoga.

Breathing plays an important role in prolonging human life. Therefore, practice Pranayama regularly.

A rabbit that breathes very rapidly does not live very long. Practice rhythmic breathing and deep breathing. There are detailed practices in Yoga for cleansing of the food-tube (Dhauti) and the stomach, as simple and effective as cleansing of the teeth. There are methods in Yoga (Trataka) for strengthening the eyesight and cleansing the nose.

People who suffer from overweight, constipation or dyspepsia will specially find this Yoga-practice very useful.

Through the practice of Yoga, the evolution of man is quickened. What he can gain in hundreds of births, he can gain in one birth through the practice of Yoga, and attain final emancipation. He can attain longevity and attain perfect health. He can compress in one life the experiences of several hundreds of births.

He who practices Basti or Yoga-enema never suffers from constipation and other abdominal disorders.

Perfection In Yoga

A Yogi can switch his life-currents, to and from the senses. He takes the Prana and the mind to the Sahasrara or the thousand-petaled lotus at the crown of the head. He enters into Samadhi. He is dead to the world. He experiences superconsciousness or Nirvikalpa Samadhi. He is in blissful union with the Lord.

Savikalpa Samadhi is subject to time and change. There is Triputi, the seer, sight and seen; or knower, knowledge and knowable. There is some link with Prakriti or matter. Savikalpa Samadhi cannot give the final emancipation. This is also an obstacle to Nirvikalpa Samadhi. The aspirant gets false contentment and stops his meditation or Sadhana. Hence this is an obstacle to the final or higher realization. Nirvikalpa Samadhi alone can burn all Samskaras and Vasanas *in toto*. Savikalpa Samadhi cannot destroy all Samskaras and Vasanas. In Savikalpa Samadhi the life-force or Prana of the Yogi is withdrawn from the body. The body appears to be dead, motionless and rigid. Breathing is suspended. He is aware of his bodily condition or suspended breath.

Nirvikalpa or Nirbija Samadhi is timeless, changeless. This is the highest state of Samadhi.

Double Consciousness

In Nirvikalpa Samadhi, the Yogi's consciousness merges with the absolute consciousness. There is no bodily fixation. In his ordinary waking consciousness, even in the midst of worldly duties, he is in communion with the supreme consciousness. He has double-consciousness.

The crow has one eyeball, but two sockets. It turns the eyeballs, now to one socket and afterwards to the other socket. Even so, the Yogi has double-consciousness.

Wise Guidance For Sure Success

The practice of Yoga should be gradual and step-by-step. Extremes are to be avoided. No sudden and violent methods should be employed. Common sense is an essential part of Yoga. Boldness is also equally essential.

Fickle-mindedness will not do on the path of Yoga. Vacillation and oscillation will retard progress and result in stagnation.

Reflect gradually and choose a method; choose a method and stick to it and persevere in it continuously. This Nishtha is necessary.

A man who digs a well should not dig a foot here, a foot there, a few feet in another place and then a fourth. If he does this, he will not find water even after digging in fifty places. Once a spot is chosen, he must dig on and on in the same place and lo, he will reach the water. Even so in

Yoga, one teacher, one path, one method, one master, one idea and one-pointed faith and devotion—all the above make up the secret of success in spiritual life.

Practice Of Yoga Asanas

1. The practice of Yoga Asanas helps to prevent disease and maintain a high standard of health, vigor and vitality. It cures many diseases.

2. It is conducive to higher intellectual and spiritual attainment and provides a co-ordinated system of health for all people.

3. There are as many Asanas as there are living creatures.

4. Siddha, Padma, Svastika, Sukha—are the four chief meditation-postures.

5. Sirshasana, Sarvangasana, Halasana, Paschimottanasana—confer wonderful health and cure many diseases.

6. The practice of Asanas is always accompanied by Pranayama and Japa of Mantra.

7. Moderation in diet and observance of Brahmacharya are necessary for realizing the maximum benefits of the practice of Asanas. A Yogi should always avoid fear, anger, laziness, too much sleep or walking, and too much food or fasting.

8. Regularity in the practice of Asanas is of paramount importance.

9. Lakhs of people have derived real benefit from the practice of Yoga Asanas.

10. Even in Europe and America, many have taken to the practice of Yoga Asanas.

11. Several Schools of Yoga in the West and India, Hong Kong, Indonesia, Australia, Denmark, Holland, show a record to prove the therapeutic value of the Asanas.

12. I have written several books on Yoga Asanas: 1. Yoga Asanas, 2. Hatha Yoga, 3. Yogic Home Exercises, 4. Radiant Health Through Yoga, 5. Practical Guide to Students of Yoga; and a number of other books like 1. Easy Steps to Yoga, 2. Yoga in Daily Life, 3. Practical Lessons in Yoga, etc., contain lessons in Yoga Asanas and Pranayama.

13. This system costs nothing. It is inexpensive. It is simple. It is specially suited for the people of the whole world at large.

14. Even women can practice it with great advantage to themselves. Irrespective of age, all can join in the practice of Yoga Asanas.

15. The benefit of Yoga Asanas should be made available to every family in the whole world. Doctors' bills can be saved.

16. Ethical culture, practice of divine virtues, a rigorous discipline of the mind, spiritual culture and meditation are also very necessary for attaining integral perfection. Asanas and Pranayamas are only a part of Yoga.

FINIS

GLOSSARY

ABHYASA—Spiritual practice. Abhyasin—
Practitioner. Acharya—Preceptor; Teacher.
Adhara—Foundation; base which supports.
Adhikarin—Qualified person. Adhyatmic—
Pertaining to Atman. Agni—Fire.

Ahankara—Egoism.
Ajna Chakra—Spiritual center at the eyebrows.
Ajnana—Ignorance.
Akasa—Ether.
Akhanda—Unbroken.
Anahata Chakra—Cardiac plexus.
Ananda—Bliss; happiness; comfort.
Antahkarana—Fourfold internal organs, viz., Manas, Chitta,
Buddhi and Ahankara.
Anubhava—Experience.
Asana—Seat; posture.
Avidya—Ignorance.

BAHIH—Outward; external.
Basti—The purificatory exercise for congested bowels.
Bhakta—Devotee.
Bhakti—Devotion.
Bhava—Feeling. Bheda—
Difference; piercing.
Bhrumadhya—The space between the eyebrows.
Bhuta Siddhi—Control over elements.
Brahmachari—Celibate. Brahmacharya—
Celibacy.
Brahmamuhurta—The period from 3 to 6 a.m. intended for
Yoga—Abhyasa.

Brahmarandhra—An aperture in the crown of the head.

CHAITANYA—Consciousness. Chakras—
Spiritual centers in Sushumna Nadi.
Chandra-Nadi—Moon-flow; another name for Ida.
Chit—Knowledge.
Chitta—Consciousness.

DANA—Charity.
Darshana—Interview.
Deha—Physical body.
Dharana—Concentration.
Dhauti—The exercise for cleaning the stomach.
Diksha—Initiation.
Dosha—Fault; impurity.
Drishti—Vision.
Duhkha— Misery; pain.
Dvesha—Hatred; repulsion.

GRIHASTHA—Householder.
Granthi—Knot.
Gulma—Chronic gastritis.
Guru—Spiritual preceptor.

ICCHA—Desire.
Ida—The Nadi that runs on the left side of Sushumna.
Indriyas—Senses.

JADA—Insentient; lifeless.
Jada Kriya—Physical exercise.
Japa—Repetition of a Mantra.
Jaya—Mastery. Jiva—
Individual soul.
Jnana-Indriyas—Five organs or senses of Knowledge. viz.,

ear, skin, eye, tongue and nose.

KAIVALYA—Isolation. Kama—
Passion, desire. Kanda—The
source of all Nadis.
Karma-Indriyas—Five organs of action, viz., speech, hands,
legs, genitals and anus.
Karma—Action; duty. Kaya—
body. Kaya-Sampat—Perfection of
body. Krama—Order.

Kripa—Grace.
Kriya—Physical action or exercises.
Krodha—Anger. Kumbhaka—
Retention of breath.
Kundalini—The mysterious power in the body.

LAKSHYA—Object of concentration.
Laya—Dissolution.

MADHYAMA—Middle; center.
Manana—Reflection or concentration.
Manas—Mind.
Mandala—Region.
Manipura—Solar plexus situated at the navel.
Mantra—Holy words.
Matsarya—Envy; jealousy. Maya—
Illusive power; veiling Shakti.
Mada—Arrogance; pride.
Mitahara—Moderation of diet.
Moha—Attachment; infatuated love.
Moksha—Liberation; emancipation.
Mouna—Vow of silence.
Mrityunjaya—Conqueror of death.

Mukti—Final beatitude.
Mula—Origin; root; base.
Muladhara Chakra—The spiritual center at the base of the spinal column.

NABHI—Navel. Nada—
Anahata Sound.
Nadi—Astral tube that carries Prana. Nasikagra Drishti—Vision at the tip of the nose.
Nauli—Purificatory exercise of abdominal region.
Neti—The exercise for cleaning the nostrils.
Nididhyasana—Profound meditation. Nirguna—
Formless; without attributes. Nishkama Karma—
Disinterested work. Nishtha—Fixity; steadiness.

Nivritti Marga—Path of renunciation.
Niyama—Religious rules; second step in Yoga.

OJAS—Spiritual energy.
Oordhvareto-Yogi—The Yogi in whom the seminal energy flows upwards.

PADMA—Lotus; Chakra; a name for the plexus.
Parama—Supreme.
Pingala—The Nadi that runs on the right side of Sushumna Nadi.
Poorna—Full.
Prakriti—Nature; undifferentiated matter.
Prana—Vital energy. Pranayama—
Regulation of breath.
Pratyahara—Withdrawing the senses from objects.
Pratyakshatva—Direct perception.
Prema—Divine love.
Prerana—Inner goading.

Puraka—Inhalation.

RAGA—Attachment.
Rajas—Passion; motion.
Rajasic—Passionate.
Rechaka—Exhalation.
Rupa—Form.

SADHAKA—Spiritual aspirant.
Sadhana—Spiritual practice.
Saguna—With form.
Sahasrara—The spiritual center at the head.
Sakshatkara—Direct perception. Sama—
Equal; balanced state of mind. Samadhi—
Superconscious state.
Samsara Chakra—Wheel of death and birth.
Samskara—Impression. Sankalpa—
Formative will; determination. Sattva—
Purity.
Sattvic—Pure. Satyam—
Truth; Brahman. Shakti—
Power.
Shat-Karmas—Six purificatory exercises of Hatha Yoga, viz.,
Dhauti, Basti, Neti, Nauli, Trataka and Kapalabhati.
Siddhas—Perfected Yogins.
Siddhi—Perfection; psychic power.
Sindur—Vermilion. Sparsha—
Touch; feeling. Sraddha—Faith.
Sravana—Hearing of Srutis.
Sthula—Physical; gross. Sukha—
Happiness; comfortable.
Sukshma—Astral; subtle.

Surya Nadi—Another name for Pingala.

Sutra—Aphorism.
Svara Sadhana—Regulation of breath.

TAMAS—Inertia; darkness.
Tamasic—Dull; lazy. Tattva—
Elements; faculty. Titiksha—
Forbearance. Trataka—Gazing at a
particular spot.
Trikala-Jnani—One who knows the past, present and
future.
Trishna—Craving.
Triveni—The place where three holy rivers meet.
Tushti—Satisfaction.

UNMANI AVASTHA—Mindless state of Yogins.
Uttama—Qualified person.

VAIRAGYA—Renunciation; dispassion.
Vajra—Adamantine; firm. Vak—
Speech.
Vasana—Impression of action that remains in the mind.
Virya—Seminal power; energy.
Vishuddha—Laryngeal plexus at the base of the throat.
Vritti—Mental function.

YAMA—The first step in Yoga.
Yatra—Pilgrimage.
Yoga—Superconscious state; union with Paramatma.
Yogic—Pertaining to Yoga.
Yogin—One who is devoted to Yoga.
Yukti—Common—sense.

"Know Thyself – The Empowering Truth of Self-Realization" (ISBN: 1497325161)

by **Lateef Terrell Warnick**

"WHO AM I?"

is the most important question in life you'll ever ask yourself! Yet many will go to their graves without ever finding a concrete answer to this question. There is one purpose to life and that is to come to **"Know Thyself!"**

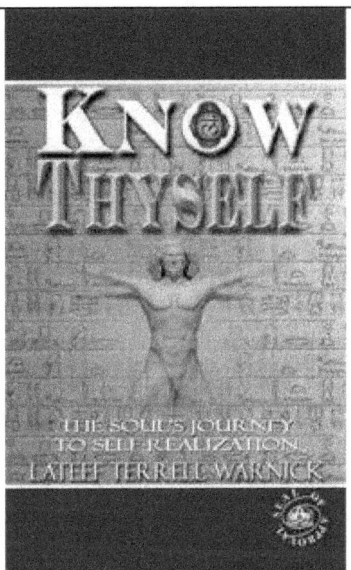

One's inner search brings the awareness and direct experience of Spirit. This is accomplished through three phases of Evolution, Experience and Enlightenment.

Evolution: The Book of Genesis symbolically represents how the world comes into being. The formless Spirit mystically descends, taking form, within creation.

Experience: Everything that we experience in this world of duality is what we call life. Through infinite possibilities, we make choices and are intended to grow and evolve but where are we going?

Enlightenment: Many take the Book of Revelation to mean "Armageddon" thus feeding fear of the end of the world. But what if hidden within these pages were secrets towards man's spiritual enlightenment?

Published by **1 S.O.U.L. Publishing**. Purchase at all major retailers like Amazon, Barnes & Noble & Books-a-Million for just $14.99 or directly at www.selfawakened.com for just $12.99 plus shipping & handling.

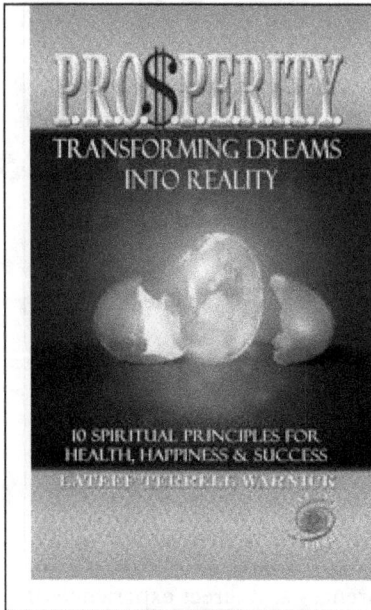

Most are familiar with the concept of karma, you reap what you sow, what goes around comes around and so on. This isn't your "bubble gum" metaphysics. This book was written for the sincere Truth Seeker that places Self-Realization first and foremost. Upon finding the Eternal treasure within, lasting prosperity is a natural result and not merely a measure of your material possessions.

P.R.O.S.P.E.R.I.T.Y. –

**"PRINCIPLE REASONS OPTIMISTIC SERVICE
PRODUCES EXPONENTIAL RICHNESS INEVITABLY
THROUGH YOU!"**

Published by **1 S.O.U.L. Publishing**. Purchase at all major retailers like Amazon, Barnes & Noble & Books-a-Million for just $11.99 or directly at **www.selfawakened.com** for just $9.99 plus shipping & handling.

"To Him That Overcometh –
Reincarnation, The Law of
Karma & Self-Realization"
(ISBN: 1939199018)

by William Walker Atkinson &
Lateef Terrell Warnick

Have I been here before? The
Answer is a resounding…
"YES!"

Explore the cultural stories
from all ages on the long-
standing debate on the aspects
of reincarnation and what it
means to your own life.

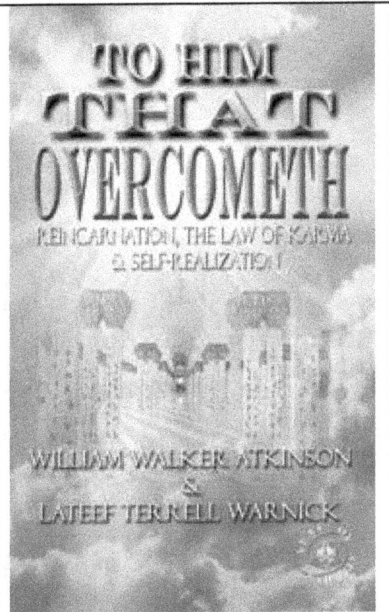

TO HIM THAT OVERCOMETH

REINCARNATION, THE LAW OF KARMA
& SELF-REALIZATION

WILLIAM WALKER ATKINSON
&
LATEEF TERRELL WARNICK

This classic book explores the concept of life and death and the
reincarnation of the soul through many lifetimes experiencing all
the impacts of the Law of Karma and cause and effect!

This book examines those beliefs from the earliest races,
Egyptians, Chaldeans, Jews, Christians and Hindus to the
present day New Agers, Yogis and Mystics. Science has already
proven that energy is never created nor destroyed, only
transformed. Likewise, the Consciousness that gives rise to life
may appear in many forms through many incarnations but the
essence of the soul is eternal without beginning nor end.

Published by **1 S.O.U.L. Publishing**. Purchase at all major
retailers like Amazon, Barnes & Noble & Books-a-Million for
just $12.95 or directly at **www.selfawakened.com** for just $10.95
plus shipping & handling.

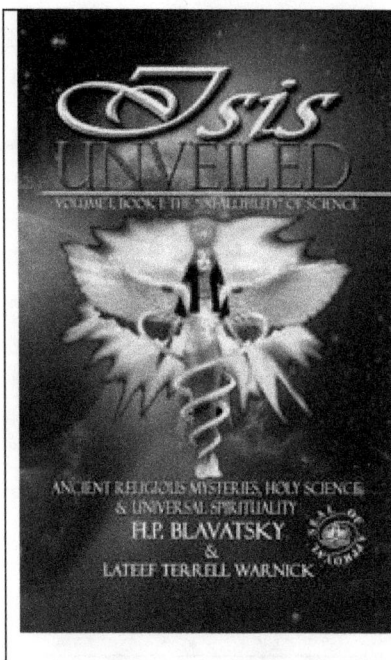

"**Isis Unveiled** – Ancient Religious Mysteries, Holy Science & Universal Spirituality"

(Volume I, Books I & II)

(ISBN: 1939199042 & 1939199077)

by **H.P. Blavatsky &
Lateef Terrell Warnick**
"Does God Really Exist"?

This is a question that has been asked since the beginning of time and probably will not be answered into the individual comes face to face with the Truth!

However, if a critical examination on the subject matter is what you're looking for then there probably is no better source than **"Isis Revealed."** This book goes in depth to explore man's place in the world, how we all relate to one another and what connects us all. For the mystic, that answer is undeniably that we are all part of One Source, One Essence and One Spirit.

Ultimately, it is the yogi who tells us that to the disbeliever there will never be substantial enough evidence to convince the doubter. However, for those who aren't merely skeptics but have a sincere thirst for Truth, then only by going within will you ever be quenched! Isis Unveiled is the rapid river leading you to the water within… *it is up to you to drink!*

Published by **1 S.O.U.L. Publishing**. Purchase at all major retailers like Amazon, Barnes & Noble & Books-a-Million for just $14.99 or directly at www.selfawakened.com for just $12.99 plus shipping & handling.

9 781939 199133